CRITICAL CARE OF THE CHILD

DEVELOPMENTS IN CRITICAL CARE MEDICINE AND ANESTHESIOLOGY

Prakash, O. (ed.): Applied Physiology in Clinical Respiratory Care. 1982. ISBN 90-247-2662-X.

McGeown, Mary G.: Clinical Management of Electrolyte Disorders. 1983. ISBN 0-89838-559-8.

Scheck, P.A., Sjöstrand, U.H., and Smith, R.B. (eds.): Perspectives in High Frequency Ventilation. 1983. ISBN 0-89838-571-7.

Stanley, T.H., and Petty, W.C. (eds.): New Anesthetic Agents, Devices and Monitoring Techniques. 1983. ISBN 0-89838-566-0.

Prakash, O. (ed.): Computing in Anesthesia and Intensive Care. 1983. ISBN 0-89838-602-0.

Stanley, T.H., and Petty, W.C. (eds.): Anesthesia and the Cardiovascular System. 1984. ISBN 0-89838-626-8.

Van Kleef, J.W., Burm, A.G.L., and Spierdijk, J. (eds.): Current Concepts in Regional Anaesthesia. 1984. ISBN 0-89838-644-6.

Prakash, O. (ed.): Critical Care of the Child. 1984. ISBN 0-89838-661-6.

CRITICAL CARE OF THE CHILD

edited by

O. PRAKASH, MD

Thoraxcentrum
Academic Hospital Dijkzigt
Erasmus University
Rotterdam
The Netherlands

1984 **MARTINUS NIJHOFF PUBLISHERS**
a member of the KLUWER ACADEMIC PUBLISHERS GROUP
BOSTON / DORDRECHT / LANCASTER

Distributors

for the United States and Canada: Kluwer Academic Publishers, 190 Old Derby Street, Hingham, MA 02043, USA
for the UK and Ireland: Kluwer Academic Publishers, MTP Press Limited, Falcon House, Queen Square, Lancaster LA1 1RN, England
for all other countries: Kluwer Academic Publishers Group, Distribution Center, P.O. Box 322, 3300 AH Dordrecht, The Netherlands

Library of Congress Cataloging in Publication Data

Main entry under title:

Critical care of the child.

(Developments in critical care medicine and anesthesiology)
Papers presented at the Second International Symposium on "Applied Physiology in Critical Care with Emphasis on Children," held in Aruba in 1983.
Includes index.
1. Pediatric intensive care--Congresses. 2. Child development--Congresses. 3. Infants--Diseases-- Congresses. I. Prakash, Omar. II. International Symposium on "Applied Physiology in Critical Care with Emphasis on Children" (2nd : 1983 : Aruba) III. Title: Applied physiology in critical care with emphasis on children. IV. Series: Developments in critical care medicine and anaesthesiology. [DNLM: 1. Child Development--congresses. 2. Critical Care-- in infancy & childhood--congresses. 3. Neonatology-- congresses. WS 366 C9333 1983]
RJ370.C745 1984   618.92'0028   84-8146

ISBN-13: 978-94-009-6038-1   e-ISBN-13: 978-94-009-6036-7
DOI: 10.1007/978-94-009-6036-7

Illustration cover: adapted from the work of Dr. Lynne Reid.

Copyright

Table of contents

Preface

This volume represents a review of recent work presented by eminent scientists at the Second International Symposium on 'Applied Physiology in Critical Care with Emphasis on Children' at Aruba, Netherlands Antilles, November 28 – 2 December, 1983.

We are grateful to the keynote speakers who accepted our invitation and completed their chapters in time for the press.

I must thank the Government of Aruba, the Tourist Office of Aruba, Mr Frank Croes and Mr Betico Croes for their support and generosity for organizing this symposium.

My sincere thanks go to Mr Rory Arends, Lucy Arends, Simon Meij and Norma van Toornburg for their untiring efforts and cooperation.

Omar Prakash, MD

List of contributors

Bryan, A.Ch., MB, BS, PhD, FRCP (C), The Hospital for Sick Children, 555 University Avenue, Toronto, Ontario, Canada M5G 1X8

Bryan, H., MD, Department of Pediatrics, Room 1241, Mount Sinai Hospital and The Hospital for Sick Children, University of Toronto, Ontario, Canada M5G 1X5
co-authors: A.L. Campbell, Y. Zarfin, M. Groenveld, P. Duffty

Enhorning, G., MD, University of Toronto, Toronto Western Hospital, 399 Bathurst Street, Toronto, Ontario, Canada M5T 2S8

Gross, I., MD, Perinatal Medicine, Yale University School of Medicine, P.O. Box 3333, New Haven, CT 06510, USA

Jobe, A., MD, Neonatal Intensive Care Unit, Harbor-UCLA Medical Center, UCLA School of Medicine, 1000 W. Carson Street, Torrance, CA 90509, USA

Jones, M.D., Jr., MD, Department of Pediatrics, Eudowood Neonatal Division, The Johns Hopkins University School of Medicine, Baltimore, MD 21205, USA

Milic-Emili, J., MD, Meakins-Christie Laboratories, McGill University, 3775 University Street, Montreal, Quebec, Canada H3A 2B4

Okken, A., MD, Division of Neonatology, Department of Pediatrics, State University, University Hospital, Oostersingel 59, 9713 EZ Groningen, The Netherlands

Orlowski, J.P. MD, Pediatric and Surgical Intensive Care Unit, Cleveland Clinic Foundation, 9500 Euclid Avenue, Cleveland, OH 44106, USA

Rabinovitch, M., MD, The Hospital for Sick Children, 555 University Avenue, Toronto, Ontario, Canada M5G 1X8

Steward, D.J., MD, FRCP (C), The Hospital for Sick Children, 555 University Avenue, Toronto, Ontario, Canada M5G 1X8

Svenningsen, N.W., MD, Department of Paediatrics, University Hospital Lund, S-221 85 Lund, Sweden

Swyer, P.R., MA, MB, FRCP (C), DCH, The Hospital for Sick Children, 555 University Avenue, Toronto, Ontario, Canada M5G 1X8

Versmold, H.T., MD, Division of Neonatology, Department of Gynecology and Obstetrics, Klinikum Grosshadern der Ludwig-Maximilians-Universität

München, Marchionistrasse 15, D-8000 München 70, Federal Republic of Germany

Wagner, P.D., MD, Section of Physiology M-023, School of Medicine, University of California San Diego, La Jolla, CA 92093, USA

1. NUTRITION, GROWTH AND METABOLISM IN THE NEWBORN

P.R. SWYER

INTRODUCTION

An understanding of the physiology of metabolism, nutrition and growth in the newborn infant and especially of the implications of pathological deviations in the very low birth weight or sick neonate is of the greatest importance to management directed at intact survival.

METABOLIC COMPARISON WITH THE ADULT

Fluid and energy intake

At best, the healthy newborn infant (and his physician) are faced with a gigantic task of gourmandise in the first few months of life. At worst, i.e., during acute illness, this task becomes even more formidable because of pathological constraints on intake in the face of increased catabolic demands. Consider that the adult, if he had to drink in proportion to the newborn's weight, would need to engulf 14 liters per day, compared with his usual 1–2 liters. This is, proportionately to body weight, 7–10 times as much fluid.

The energy intake required for metabolic maintenance for the newborn is increased 2–3 fold/kg compared with the adult (i.e, 50–60 cf 20 kcal/kg/d). On top of this maintenance requirement is that for growth which is obviously lacking for the adult. Growth necessitates an approximate doubling of the energy for maintenance (Figure 1) to over 100 kcal/kg/d.

The effects of growth on body composition. Implied macronutrient requirement

Table 1 shows the body composition of the infant at birth weights of 1 kg, 2 kg and 3.5 kg, corresponding to postconceptional ages of 28 weeks, 35 weeks and 40 weeks respectively (1, 2). In comparison with the adult, the fetus of 1 kg or less is little more than a bag of water (86%) lightly tinted with protein (8%). The fetus is

TOTAL ENERGY INTAKE

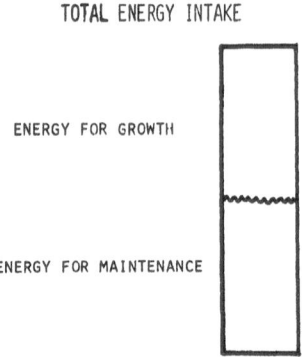

ENERGY FOR GROWTH

ENERGY FOR MAINTENANCE

Figure 1. The partition of energy intake is approximately equal for maintenance and growth.

virtually devoid of fat (0.1%) and contains only a smattering of carbohydrate (0.045%). The total energy content is 460 kcal, mostly proteinaceous. The 2 kg infant, with the benefit of a further 7 weeks' gestation, has accumulated an additional 145 grams of protein and has developed a fat organ of 100 grams The total energy content is 1900 kcal with 970 kcal from nonprotein sources, mostly fat. The term infant has accumulated a furher 160 grams of protein and 460 grams of fat and now has a total energy content of 6950 kcals, 70% derived from fat. These represent average figures for normally grown infants. The paucity of energy, especially fat reserves of the infant by comparison with the adult is evident and justifies the urgency of neonatal macronutrient repletion.

Table 1. Body composition of infants weighing 1, 2 and 3.5 kg cf adult.

	28 weeks	35 weeks	40 weeks	Adult
Weight (g)	1000	2000	3500	70000
Water	860	1620	2400	42000
Protein	85	230	390	12000
Fat	10	100	560	15300
CHO	4.5	9	34	700
Total kcal	460	1900	6950	188500
Nonprotein kcal	110	970	5350	140500
MMR kcal	50	106	186	1400
MMR/Nonprotein kcal	1:2	1:9	1:29	1:100

MMR = minimal metabolic rate.
Modified by Sinclair from data of Widdowson and Spray (1), with additions.

PARTITIONAL USE OF ENERGY INTAKE

By combining balance studies with computerized indirect calorimetry, we have

3

partitioned the use of the energy intake as shown in Figure 2 (3).

After birth there is a steady increase in food intake which is accompanied by a rise in metabolic rate.

Once stabilization has occurred for the very low birth weight infant at about 3 weeks of age, this partition is proportioned as shown in Figure 3. Energy losses, mostly as stool fat, account for 12%; energy for maintenance 32%, activity 3%, energy for tissue synthesis 8%, and energy stored in new tissue, almost half of intake at 46%.

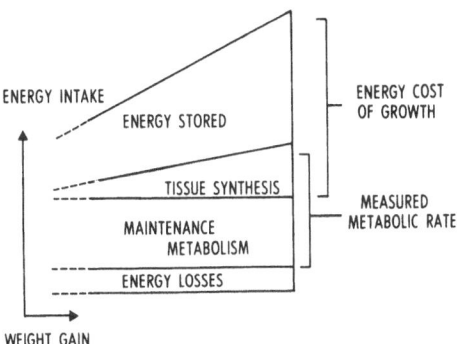

Figure 2. Diagrammatic representation of changes in energy intake and energy utilization with time and increase in body weight.

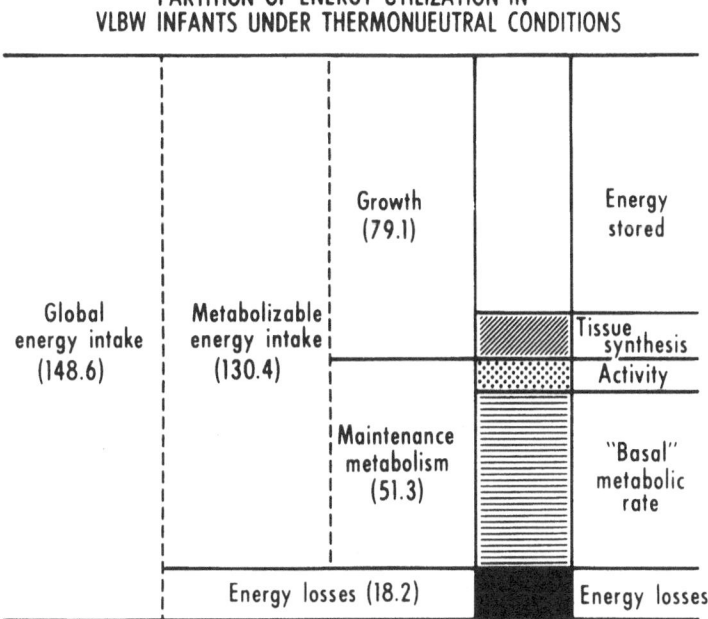

Figure 3. *n* = 22; Reichman et al. (3)

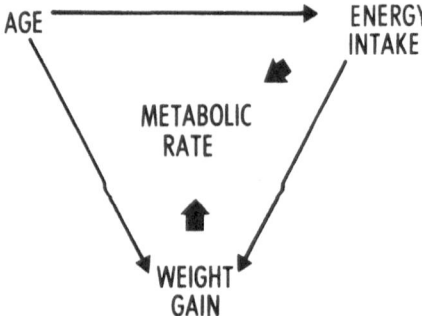

Figure 4. Diagrammatic representation of the interdependence of age, energy intake, weight gain and metabolic rate.

INFLUENCE OF GROWTH ON METABOLIC RATE

The increase in metabolic rate after birth requires explanation. It does not appear to be simply a maturational effect of age, but is a combined and interdependent effect of age, level of energy intake, and growth (Figure 4). Increasing energy intake with age engenders tissue growth and weight gain, entailing increased energy expenditure (4).

The increase in metabolic rate is closely related to the so-called thermic effect of food, or specific dynamic action. This is a manifestation of the exothermic

Table 2. Heat production from energy deposition and conversion of the principle nutrients

Biochemical transformations involved in energy deposition[a]	Energy cost of conversion kcal/g end product	Percentage of initial energy lost during transformation
Fat into fat[b]: triglyceride → free fatty acids → triglyceride	0.095	1
Carbohydrate into fat[c]: 14 glucose + 12 O_2 → tripalmitylglycerate + 33 CO_2 + 21 ATP	1.419	15
Protein into fat[d]: 21 amino acids + 48.3 O_2 → tripalmitylglycerate + 36 CO_2 + 14.4 urea	2.933	31
Protein into protein: 1 amino acid + 5 ATP → 1 peptide	0.648	15
Glucose into glycogen[e]	0.376	9

[a] Calculations based on molecular weights of 806, 162 and 110 and the heat contents of 9.46, 4.18 and 4.32 kcal/g for triglyceride, carbohydrate and protein. ATP is assumed to be formed from dietary carbohydrate at a rate of 37 mole/mole glucose.
[b] Assuming a requirement of 6 ATP per mole triglyceride.
[c] Assuming conversion as described in McGilvery (68); RQ = 2.75.
[d] Assuming conversion via glucose and ketones as described in McGilvery (68); RQ = 0.75.
[e] Assuming a requirement of 3 ATP per mole glycogen.
Modified from Millward and Garlick (69).
By permission from Heim (70).

reactions involved in the reorganization of the ingested food molecules into new tissue, notably tissue protein (Table 2).

One could envisage a process akin to that shown on the next slide (Figure 5) taking place. Metabolic heat is produced by maintenance of body functions with an additional component resulting from continuous muscle protein net synthesis. After each meal, new protein is synthesized, mainly in the liver, for transport to the periphery and is accompanied by a postprandial thermic effect. These synthetic processes will increase with the level of food intake and account for the postnatal increase in metabolic rate. Of course, other metabolic processes than net protein synthesis will also contribute to the postprandial thermic effect (Table 2).

Support for the concept of the stimulative effect of food intake on metabolic rate comes from several sources. Scopes and his co-workers (5) measured the oxygen uptake of two groups of low birth weight infants, in 1966 when neonatal feeding was restricted, and again in 1974 after neonatal feeding had been liberalized (6). There was an increase in the second period. Studies of the rates of oxygen uptake in the refeeding of malnourished infants by Ashworth (7) has also shown a proportionate increase in $\dot{V}O_2$ to rate of weight gain. Our own studies (4) of increase in metabolic rate with age show also parallel increases of energy intake and rate of weight gain (Figure 6). There is a linear relationship between energy intake and metabolic rate (Figure 7), and between weight gain and metabolic rate (Figure 8). Each gram of weight gained increases the metabolic rate by 0.67 kcal.

The need to support growth by proper nutrition, even in the sick neonate, introduces a completely new dimension to their intensive care compared to the sick adult.

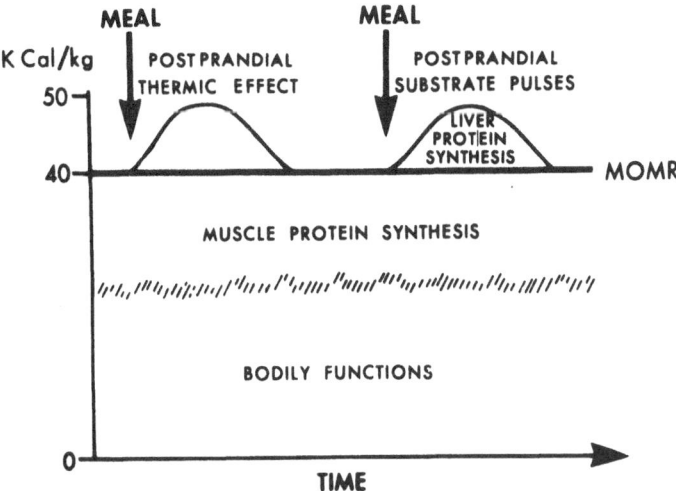

Figure 5. Diagram of energy utilization for bodily functions, muscle protein synthesis and protein synthesis in the liver giving rise to the postprandial thermic effect (specific dynamic action of food).

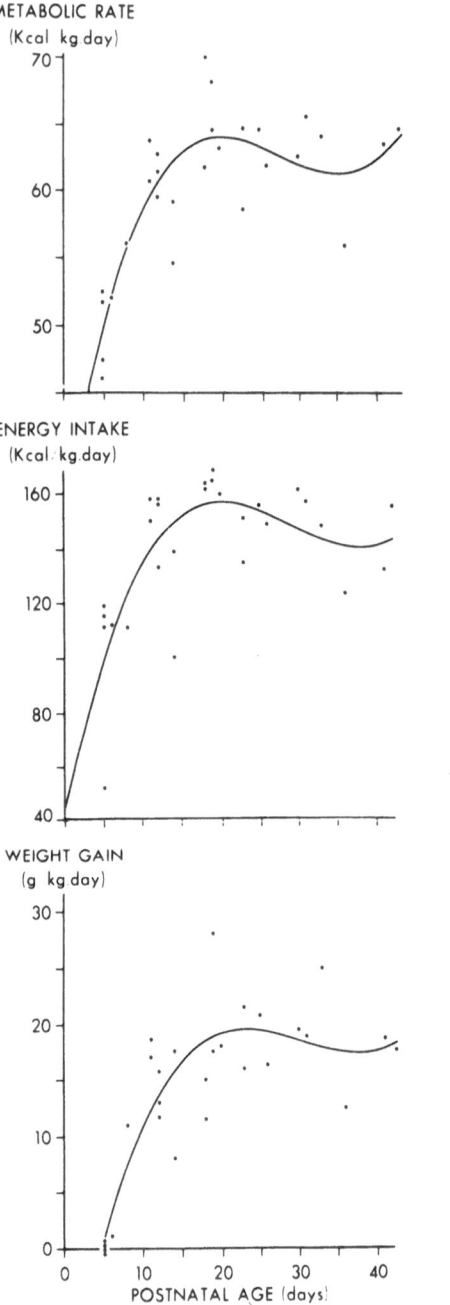

Figure 6. Polynomial regression analysis showing in 28 studies the similar pattern of lines of best fit between metabolic rate (kcal/kg/day), energy intake (kcal/kg/day) and weight gain (gm/kg/day) with increasing postnatal age (A): MR = $0.00165A^3 - 0.138A^2 + 3.56A + 35.4$; $r = 0.85$, $p<0.001$; EI = $0.00591A^3 - 0.516A^2 + 13.61A + 44.6$; $r = 0.74$, $p<0.001$; WtG = $0.00138A^3 - 0.126A^2 + 3.65A - 14.5$; $r = 0.86$, $p<0.001$. Reproduced with permission from Chessex et al. (4).

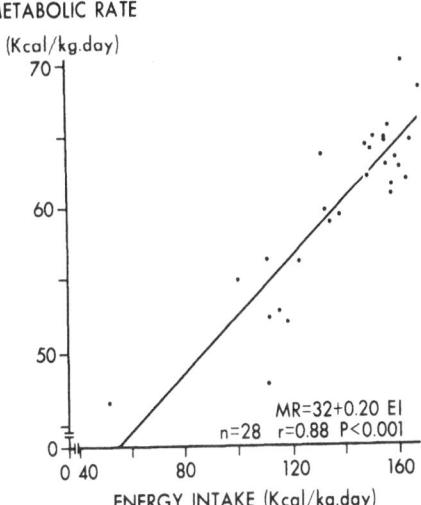

Figure 7. Relationship between metabolic (MR, kcal/kg/day) and increasing energy intake (EI, kcal/kg/day) in 28 studies: MR = 32 + 0.20 EI; $r = 0.88$, $p<0.001$. Reproduced with permission from Chessex et al. (4).

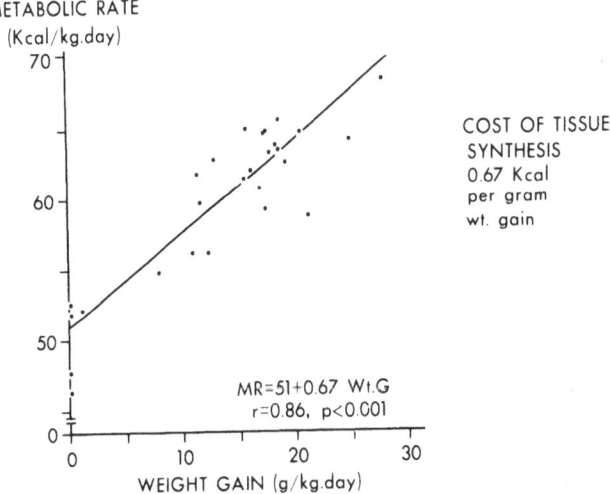

Figure 8. Relationship between metabolic rate (MR, kcal/kg/day) and weight gain (WtG, g/kg/day) in 28 studies: MR = 51 + 0.67 WtG; $r = 0.86$, $p<0.001$. Reproduced with permission from Chessex et al. (4).

Adequate nutrition is increasingly identified in the adult as important to survival. Undernutrition in the newborn adds the future menace of stunted mental and physical development to the immediate threat of compromised physiological function and death.

COMPROMISED PHYSIOLOGICAL FUNCTIONS IN THE SICK NEONATE WITH NUTRITIONAL
CONNOTATIONS

Hypoglycemia

The most obvious is neonatal hypoglycemia common in prematures, infants small
for gestational age, and postmature infants suffering from placental insufficiency.
It results from the deficient energy stores in the very low birth weight or sick
infant (Table 1).

Since the neonatal heart is dependent for energy on its glycogen reserves and
glucose catabolism rather than on fatty acid energy derivation as in the adult, the
myocardium can be compromised even to the extent of acute dilatation and
failure (8) (Figure 9A). This condition can be rapidly cured by glucose infusion
(Figure 9B). Transient myocardial ischemia in the newborn (9), though usually
developing on a postasphyxial hypoxic-ischemic basis, frequently is potentiated
by concomitant hypoglycemia. Since the brain is largely dependent on glucose for
energy, hypoglycemia may provoke serious central nervous system symptoms,
including convulsions and may have serious remote effects on brain development
and function.

Dehydration

Failure of adequate fluid intake may, in addition to deficiency of energy substrate, lead to acute or subacute dehydration, with electrolyte disturbances,
convulsions and eventual cardiorespiratory failure.

Hypothermia

Deficiency of energy intake results, especially in the very low birth weight
premature without substrate reserves, in an inability to maintain body temperature because of failure of adequate heat production with falling metabolic rate
(10).

Apnea repetens

Apnea in the low birth weight newborn appears typically on the third day of life
when meager energy reserves have been used up. Recent thinking ascribes
postnatal apnea repetens to fatigue of the muscles of respiration, stressed by the
increased work of breathing due to a soft chest wall and poor coupling between
the diaphragm and the intercostal musculature, and paucity of high oxidative type

9

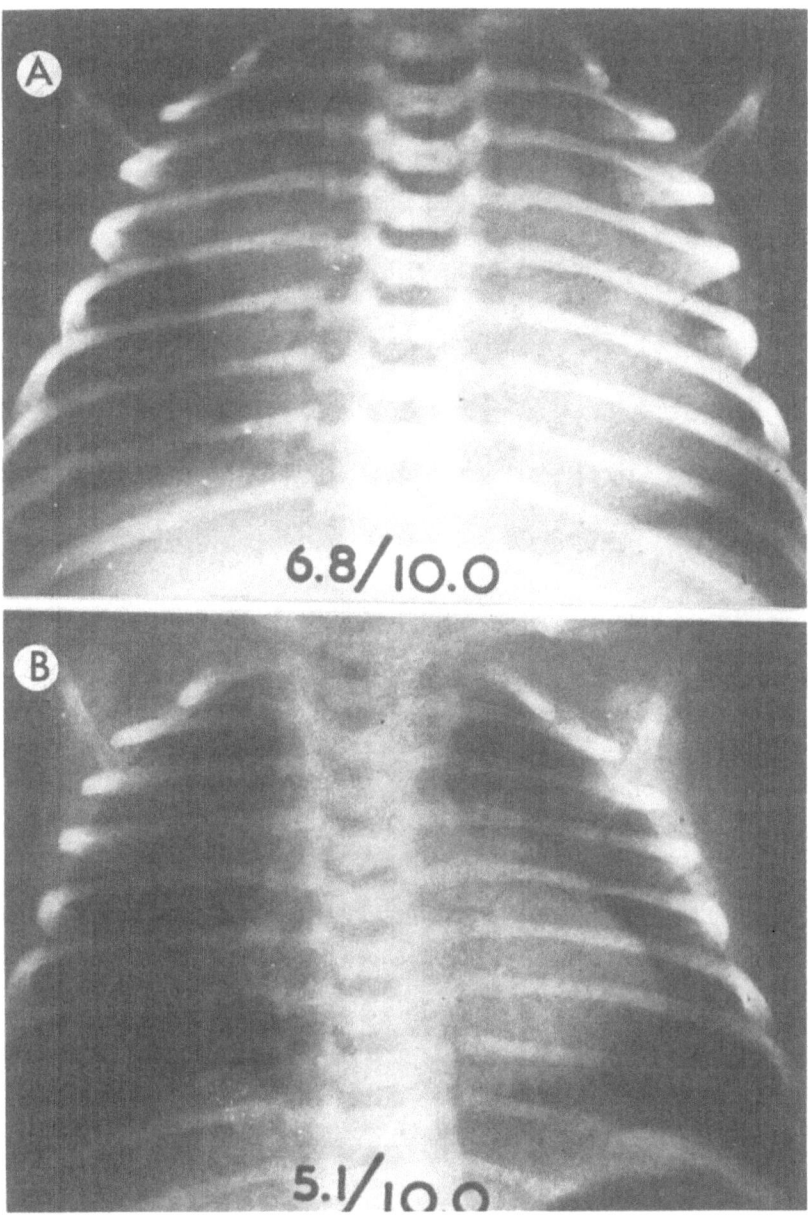

Figure 9. (A) Acute cardiac dilatation in an infant whose blood sugar was zero; (B) Return to normal size on treatment of hypoglycemia.

10

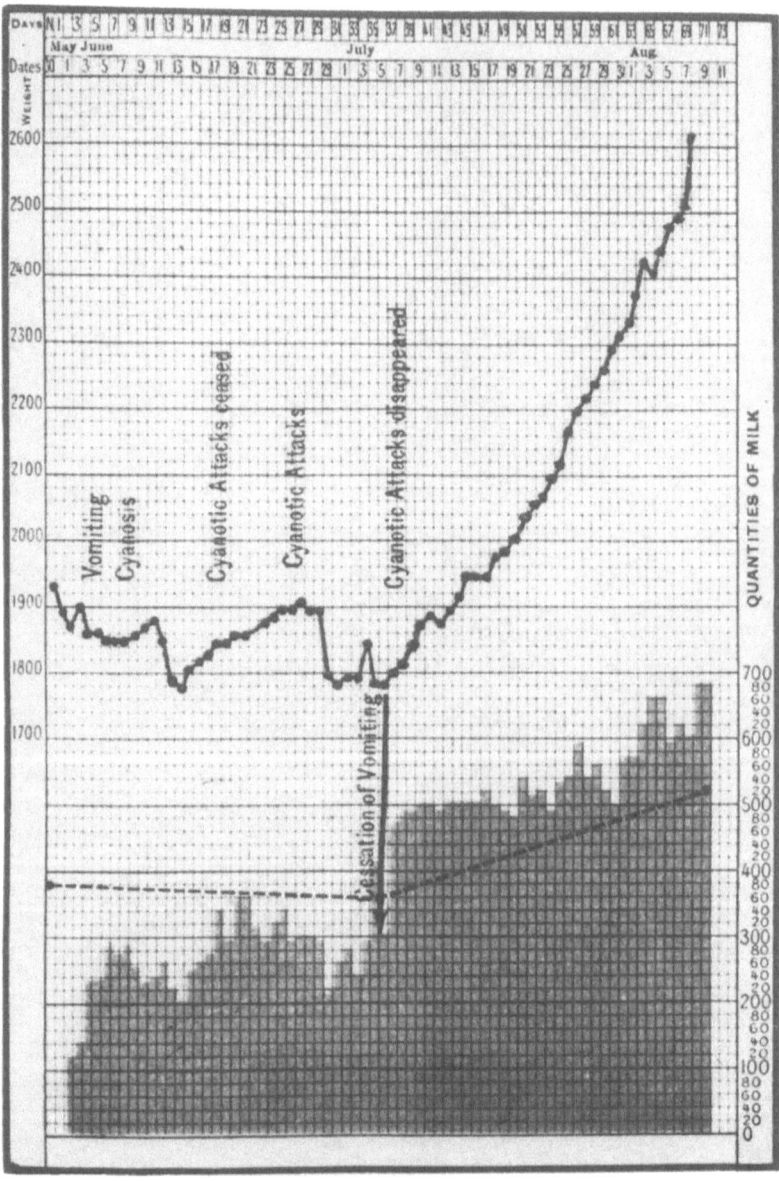

Figure 10. Cyanotic attacks in a weakling due to underfeeding. The black columns which represent the daily amount taken by the infant, do not attain the interrupted line, which indicates the minimum amount required by an infant of this weight. The attacks ceased when the infant was adequately fed. Reproduced from Budin (12).

1 fibers in the diaphragmatic muscle of the premature (11). It is also hypothesized but not yet proven, that relative substrate deficiency plays a role. Budin (12) recognized at the turn of the century that apnea was commoner in underfed infants (Figure 10). More recently, a reduction in the daily frequency of apnea has been demonstrated (13) in prematures in our clinic fed amino acid and glucose intravenously compared with those fed glucose only (Figure 11).

Essential fatty acid deficiency

Essential fatty acid deficiency has recently been recognized as having widespread adverse consequences on cellular membrane function, on myelination and brain development, and on synthesis of the prostaglandins (14). Figure 12 shows typical skin lesions in a very low birth weight infant referred to our hospital at the age of 5 days having received only glucose and electrolyte solutions since birth. Biochemical evidence of essential fatty acid deficiency was marked and the infant improved rapidly with intravenous lipid emulsion which contains approximately 60% essential fatty acids.

The sequels of essential fatty acid deficiency include:
Clinical
    Cessation of growth
    Desquamating skin rash
    Loss of hair
    Susceptibility to infection

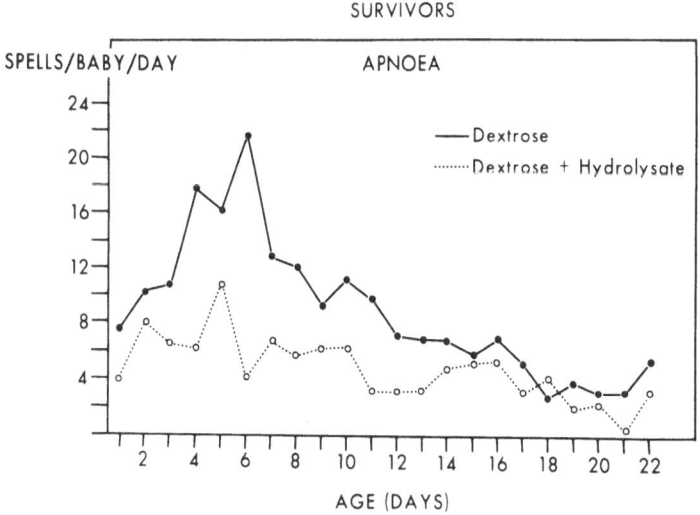

Figure 11. Frequency of apnea spells in infants receiving intravenous 10% Dextrose (●——●) and infants receiving 10% Dextrose and casein hydrolysate (○——○). Note the fewer apneic spells per baby per day in infants alimented with Dextrose and casein hydrolysate.
Reproduced with permission from Bryan et al. (13).

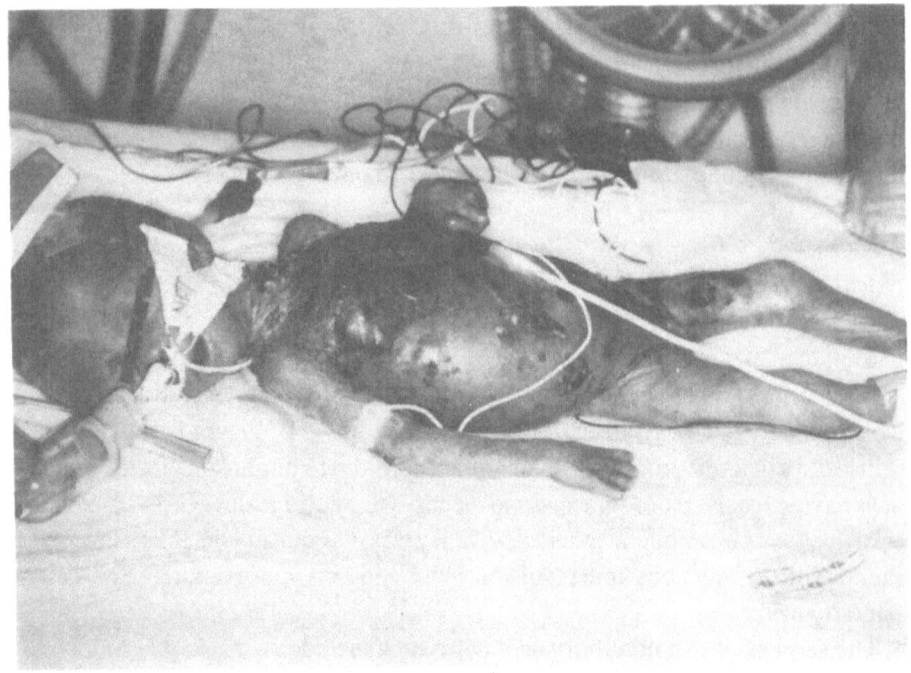

Figure 12. Baby boy Y: photograph of the skin lesions of essential acid deficiency. Reproduced with permission from Swyer (71).

    Delayed wound healing
    Thrombocytopenia
Histological
    Changes in skin, gonads, kidneys
CNS
    Retardation in cell division and growth
    Behavioral abnormalities, often irreversible and manifested in experimental animals' offspring
Physiological
    Deficiency of prostaglandin precursors
    Defects in cell membrane function
Biochemical
    Increased ratio of tri-enoic (C20:3) to tetra-enoic acids (C20:4), (15, 16) normally less than 0.4
    Decreased plasma levels of linoleic linolenic and arachidonic acids, as early as 3–4 days of life in very low birth weight infants (17)
    Decreased plasma cholestorol linoleate in LDL and HDL fractions (18, 19)

Protein (and caloric) deficiency

Deficient protein intake, which in developed countries is most frequently seen in low birth weight infants fed pooled human milk with a low protein content, results in hypoalbuminemia, edema, growth failure, and possible immunodeficiencies. The fully developed syndrome of Kwashiorkor (protein/calorie malnutrition) is seldom seen in developed countries.

Development of the gut

The development of the gut in the newborn is particularly dependent on adequate nutrition and furthermore, adequate enteral nutrition (20, 21).

Exposure of the gastrointestinal tract to nutrients exerts trophic influences on growth of intestinal villi, intestinal weight and length, and on enzyme induction in the brush border. Intestinal stasis is avoided, toxic absorption from the gut prevented, and bile stasis, excessive enterohepatic recirculation and clinical jaundice prevented.

PRACTICAL PROBLEMS IN FEEDING OF THE NEWBORN

There are therefore abundant reasons for the maintenance of adequate nutritional intake for the newborn, and especially for the sick or premature newborn. Unfortunately, there are equally abundant obstacles to the achievement of adequate nutrition. The sick or premature infant is unable to coordinate sucking, swallowing and breathing. Tube feeding is necessary with attendant dangers of bradycardia during placement, malposition of catheter, trauma or perforation of viscus and vomiting and aspiration.

Stomach capacity and gut development

Stomach capacity is very restricted at birth as shown in Table 3. Expansion of stomach volume and gut development is dependent on enteral feeding, as is the stimulation of numerous gut hormones of nutritional and metabolic importance (Table 4).

Interference with respiration

Distension of the gastrointestinal tract with milk may, by raising intra-abdominal pressure, embarrass respiration and cause a fall in FRC (22) and PaO_2, presum-

Table 3. Neonatal stomach capacity and feeding volume

Age (days)	Capacity (ml/kg birth weight)	Volume (ml/kg birth weight)
1	2	1
3	10	5
5	19	10
7	21	12–15
10	27	15–17

Table 4. Neonatal gut hormones

Hormone	Function
Gastrin	Acid output ? G.I. growth
Gastric inhibitory polypeptide	↓ Gastric secretion, motility
	↑ Insulin
Motilin	↑ G.I. motility
Secretin	Pancreatic secretion
Cholecystokinin-pancreozymin	Gall bladder contraction, Pancreatic secretion
Somatostatin	↓ Insulin
	↑ Glucagon

ably due to airway closure, atelectasis and an increase in intrapulmonary and/or interatrial shunt (Figure 13). Apnea may also be provoked.

Incompetent gastrointestinal tract

Furthermore, overloading of the gut has been implicated as one of the factors in the causation of necrotizing enterocolitis (23). Enteral feeding may be impossible because of neonatal ileus common in very low birth weight prematures, gastrointestinal malformations, or serious illness with coma or convulsions.

STRATEGY FOR THE MAINTENANCE OF NUTRITION FOR THE HIGH RISK NEONATE

Despite all these problems of enteral and parenteral feeding, the risks have to be accepted if the short- and long-term evils of malnutrition are to be avoided. In practice, a pragmatic approach based on the art of the clinically possible is necessary.

15

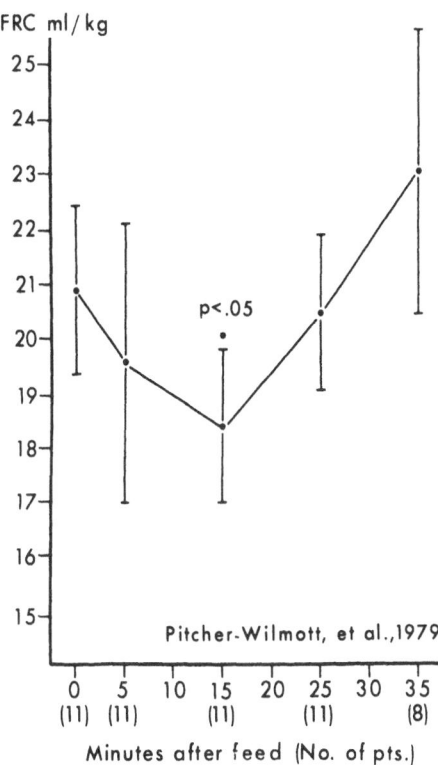

Figure 13. Reduction in functional residual capacity after feeding.
Reproduced with permission from Pitcher-Wilmott (22).

Nasogastric feeding

I prefer gastric to jejunal intubation as being easier of placement, less liable to
cause perforation and apparently of equal or greater efficacy for absorption (24).
I also prefer intermittent rather than continuous gavage feeding. Bolus feeding
seems more physiological and has the advantage of surveillance of the feeding
process by the caretaker. On occasion, however, I have found a continuous
gravity drip feed more effective in securing weight gain than conventional bolus
feeding, but such continuous drip feeding requires the closest supervision to
detect undue abdominal distension and/or regurgitation. The smallest infants
(less than 1000 g) require intermittent gavage feeding at 1–2-hr intervals. Once
weight gain is established the interval may be increased to 2–3 hr, depending on
gastric emptying time as judged by stomach aspiration prior to the feed. A residue
of more than 2–3 ml should prompt a review of volumes and feeding intervals.

Finally nonnutritive suckling by the provision of pacifiers during tube feeding
results in earlier effective nutritive suckling, better weight gain and earlier
discharge from hospital (25).

Parenteral techniques

There are very considerable technical problems associated with parenteral infusion in neonates, particularly the very low birth weight infant.

The standard technique of infusion through percutaneously placed #25 steel needles in scalp or other peripheral vein requires skill, is short-lived (15.4 ± 13.2 hr mean ± SD) (26) and may terminate in tissue infiltration and local necrosis depending on the volume and nature of the fluid extravasated.

Recently #24 gauge Teflon peripheral catheters have been found to have more than three times longer effective duration and a lower infiltration rate (26).

Many of the difficulties associated with peripheral intravenous infusion sites stem from the small and fragile nature of the veins, the minimal or no flow condition at the injection site and the irritant chemical or hyperosmolar nature of the injected fluid. In order to overcome these disadvantages, larger central veins, the umbilical, vena cavae and right atrium have been cannulated. Umbilical venous catheterization has well-recognized hazards and is consequently seldom used except for short-term cannulation at birth. However, the placement of central venous silastic catheters either percutaneously or by surgical incision and subcutaneous tunnelling to exit at a remote easy-to-manage site has increasingly been practiced (27, 28). Recently an 88% success rate has been reported for basilic or external jugular vein percutaneous placement (29) in infants less than 1000 grams in weight. These 0.635 mm external diameter silastic catheters remained functional for a mean of 24.8 ± 15.9 days. There was no associated infection or thrombosis. If these figures for reliability and freedom from complication are confirmed, the technique may well prove to be the prime choice for all intravenous therapy in high risk newborns.

The human milk controversy for the very low birth weight infant

The usual starting point for designing the diet of a very low birth weight infant is the fetal accretion rate of macro- and micronutrients (30, 31, 32). There is, however, no certainty that intrauterine rates are necessarily suitable for the extrauterine premature infant. This particularly applies to adipose tissue and body water accretion. Desirable body composition remains to be defined, but can be influenced by diet both qualitatively and quantitatively. The triglyceride composition of body fat reflects that of the dietary intake and its amount that of the gross energy and fat intake (Figure 14B).

The choices available for gastrointestinal feeding are: (a) the mother's own milk; (b) specially adapted formulas; (c) pooled mature human milk. Of these, pooled mature milk is the least desirable as it is low in protein, sodium, potassium, magnesium and calcium compared with the estimated requirements. Atkinson et al. (33, 34) have shown that the early milk contains an enhanced

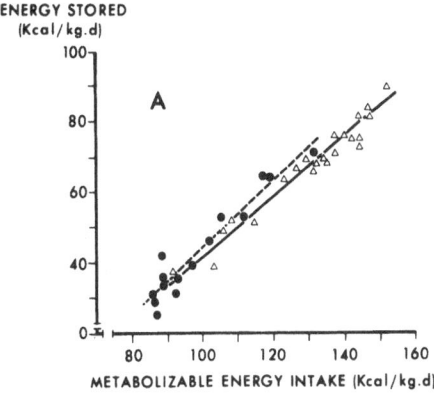

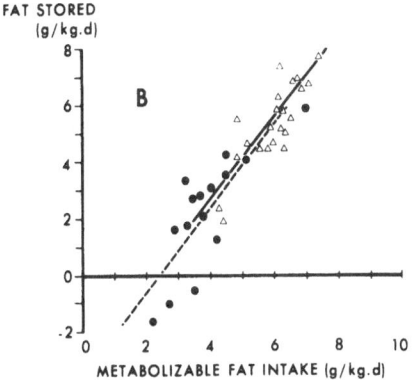

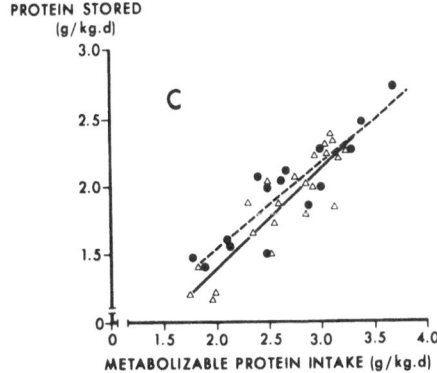

Figure 14. Linear regression of metabolizable intake versus storage of (A) energy, (B) fat and (C) protein in own mother's milk fed (solid circle), broken line) and formula fed (open triangle, solid line) infants. Note the similarity of the regressions for the two groups. The correlation coefficients ranged from 0.81–0.98 (*p*<0.001).

Reproduced with permission from Reichman et al. (42).

protein and electrolyte content more nearly satisfying estimated requirements.

Chessex et al. (35) have recently shown that very low birth weight infants fed their own mother's milk accrete protein and fat and gain in weight, head circumference and body length at approximately intrauterine rates. Similar claims have been made for the specially modified 'premature' formulas (36–41).

Our studies (42) indicate that accretion rates for energy (Figure 14A), fat (Figure 14B) and protein (Figure 14C) are linear functions of metabolizable intake. As a consequence the composition of the weight gain differs according to the composition of the dietary intake (43). For example, Figure 15 shows the

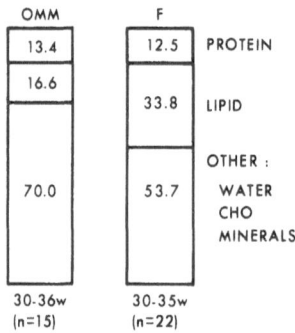

Figure 15. Comparison of the percentage composition of weight gain for infants fed their own mother's milk (OMM) (30–36 weeks postconceptional age) or formula (F) (30–35 weeks postconceptional age). Reproduced with permission from Reichman et al. (42).

higher water and lower lipid accretion of very low birth weight infants fed their own mother's milk in contrast to infants fed a calorie-dense formula (24 kcal/oz, 85 kcal/dl). At present we have insufficient evidence on which to base recommendations on desirable body composition. Infantile obesity seems to have no advantages and a possible disadvantage as a precursor of obesity in later life. Metabolizable energy intake should therefore probably be moderate and on the order of 100–110 kcal/kg/d with macronutrients and water allowances as shown in Table 5.

These requirements for macronutrients and energy appear adequately to be

Table 5. Daily water, macronutrient and metabolisable energy requirement for the newborn

	Intake/kg/d	kcal (metabolizable)
Water	150 – 200 ml	
Protein	3 g	14
Lipid	3 – 4 g	36
CHO	12 – 14 g	50
		100

fulfilled by feeding very low birth weight infants their own mother' milk at a rate of about 175 ml/kg/d (42, 44–48).

The enhanced mineral content of human preterm milk tends to disappear during the third and fourth week after birth (34). Therefore it is necessary to supplement with sodium, calcium and probably phosphorus (49, 50). The sodium supplements may be given orally as sodium bicarbonate 8.4%, 0.2 ml (0.2 mEq) every 4 hr with feeds (1.2 mEq/day) until the infant reaches a weight of 1500 grams; then 0.4 ml (0.4 mEq) q 4 hr (2.4 mEq/day) until the infant reaches a weight of 1800 grams. Oral calcium supplements should supply approximately 6 mEq/kg/d of elemental calcium of which only about 30% is actually absorbed. The total daily requirement for absorption is 3–4 mEq of elemental calcium. These supplements should be given up to a weight of 1500 grams after which the mature human milk content of 17 mEq/L suffices.

If the infant's own mother's milk is not available, the new 'special premie' formulas would now seem to be reasonable alternatives (36–41). Such formulas supply an adequate β-lactoglobulin component in a whey predominant (60/40 whey/casein) mixture. They have an enhanced content of medium-chain trig-lycerides which improves fat absorption (51, 52, 53) because they are directly absorbed in the upper small intestine and hence do not require bile salts (possibly deficient in the premature) and lipase (absent in formula, but present in human milk). They also contain modified carbohydrate, glucose or glucose polymers replacing some or all of the lactose. This replacement of lactose, based on the later development of lactase in the intestinal brush border compared with maltase and sucrase, may reduce absorption of fat, calcium and magnesium. The desir-ability of such replacement remains questionable. Most special premature for-mulas are calorie dense (84 kcal/dl, 24 kcal/oz) and may supply too much energy if volume intake is normal to high (43). However, some premie formulas are supplied at a 64 kcal/dl, 20 kcal/oz concentration. All have varying degrees of mineral supplementation, and further supplementation is usually not required. Finally, the daily intake of vitamin D should provide at least 1000 units daily for the very low birth weight infant which mandates supplementation for both human milk and formula-fed premature infants (54, 55), in order to promote normal bone mineralization.

Partial and total enteral/parenteral nutrition for the very low birth weight infant

Granted that gastrointestinal alimentation is the preferred method of nutrition for the very low birth weight infant, there are nevertheless absolute contraindica-tions. Some circumstances permit only partial satisfaction of enteral needs, thus requiring intravenous supplementation.

Indications for parenteral nutrition are usually because of the dangers of vomiting and aspiration secondary to ileus or obstruction.

When these absolute indications cease to exist, or the primary condition improves, there should be a cautious introduction of gastrointestinal feedings, usually by the nasogastric route. Parenteral volume is reciprocally reduced as gastrointestinal volume is increased according to tolerance over several days as the primary condition improves.

Initial parenteral supplementation in the very low birth weight infant is with 5 g/dl glucose in water at 80 to 100 ml/kg/24 hourly, thus supplying 4 g (16 kcal) to 5 g (20 kcal) of glucose. This intake supplies about one third of the resting requirements for energy. After the first six hours, calcium should be added at a rate of 2 mEq/kg/d. After 12–24 hr, sodium should be added by changing the infusion to 0.2% NaCl with 5 g/dl dextrose which supplies 3.4 mEq/kg of sodium when given at a rate of 100 ml/kg/d. As glucose tolerance improves after 48 hr the concentration of glucose may be raised to 10 g/dl, monitoring glycosuria, and blood glucose every 6 hr initially. The intravenous solutions are reduced as gastrointestinal feedings increase. If gastrointestinal feedings are contraindicated, total parenteral nutrition becomes urgent and a 5 g/dl dextrose, 2 g/dl amino acid solution is introduced and then the glucose concentration increased to 10 g/dl. Table 6 shows the composition of the two solutions used for prematures in the Neonatal Intensive Care Unit of the Hospital for Sick Children, Toronto.

Provided contraindications do not exist, a 10 g/dl lipid emulsion is then 'piggy backed' in at a rate of 0.5 to 1 g/kg/d, increasing gradually to 3–4 g/kg/d over the succeeding 7–14 days as indicated by monitoring of serum triglyceride levels, daily at first, and then twice weekly as tolerance is established. The serum triglyceride level should be below 100 mg/dl (56, 57). While most newborns readily metabo-

Table 6. Composition of standard solutions (per litre) - Premature Infants P5 and P10

	P5	P10
Protein G	20	20
Glucose G	50	100
Na mmol	14	14
K mmol	15	15
Cl mmol	14	14
Ca mmol	6.5	6.5
P mmol	6.0	6.0
Mg mmol	3.0	3.0
Zn μmol	14	14
Cu μmol	6.25	6.25
Mn μmol	9.0	9.0
I μmol	0.47	0.47
Cr μmol	0.048	0.048
Se μmol	0.38	0.38
Fe μmol	18	18

The amino acid source used 2% Vamin. Minerals expressed in μmoles. For patients on TPN for no longer than 4 weeks, iron at the levels shown should be included in the Standard Solution (Division of Nutrition, Hospital for Sick Children, Toronto).

lize fat as shown by fall in RQ to about 0.7 soon after birth (58) and by indirect calorimetric studies during infusion of lipid emulsion (59), the very low birth weight infant is deficient in the key enzyme lipoprotein lipase in proportion to immaturity and dysmaturity (60, 61). As a consequence, plasma clearance of chylomicrons and other lipids may be impaired. Sequels may include reduced pulmonary diffusing capacity and arterial oxygen tension with pulmonary capillary lipid deposition, potential displacement of bilirubin from serum albumin binding sites, interference with photometric measurement of serum bilirubin levels, lipid deposition in the reticuloendothelial system, leukocytes and macrophages impairing defense against infection. The use of lipid emulsions in infants with pulmonary disease; with bilirubinemia of more than 50% of the threshold level for exchange; with hepatic injury; with infection, extreme prematurity or intrauterine growth retardation is hazardous, and the advantages should be carefully weighed against the hazards. Desirable daily water and macronutrient intakes are shown in Table 5.

In most prematures, total or partial parenteral nutrition is seldom required for longer than two weeks, by which time the enteral route is sufficient and preferable, even for infants recovering from necrotizing enterocolitis providing perforation has not occurred and surgical intervention has not been required.

Total parenteral nutrition for the 'surgical' neonate

The availability of total parenteral nutrition has completely transformed the prognosis for infants with major anomalies and conditions affecting the gastrointestinal tract such as atresia, volvulus, malrotation, omphalocele and gastroschisis, especially where major resections have to be undertaken. While it is possible to maintain infants almost indefinitely on total parenteral nutrition with an afunctional gut, the prospects for normal life and growth are in practice remote where a major resection has removed the ileocecal valve and left less than 40 cm of small bowel (62). In such cases most would reject prolonged total parenteral nutrition. In all others, total parenteral nutrition has been shown to support normal life and growth over many weeks, even months, until the remaining gut can adapt. Such patients will usually be managed by central silastic catheterization (27,28).

OUTCOME AND GOALS FOR NUTRITION OF THE NEONATE: PROBLEMS IN EVALUATION, BODY COMPOSITION AND MENTAL DEVELOPMENT

The prognosis for the high risk very low birth weight newborn has improved remarkably, the mortality rate having fallen from 85% to 21% in The Hospital for Sick Children, Toronto, in the last twenty years. This improvement has been achieved because of a better understanding of the pathophysiological processes underlying disease in the fetus and newborn and the consequential introduction of new techniques of resuscitation, respiratory and other life support, neonatal anesthesia and surgery.

As a consequence, the gut and nutritional function are now prime factors in intact survival for the high risk infant.

The objective of a nutritional regimen for the high risk sick or premature neonate is to support life and a rate of growth sufficient to fulfill the individual's genetic potential.

From the environmental point of view, Widdowson and McCance (62) discussed the important concept of 'critical epochs' in development 'when the size of the animal arising from its previous plane of nutrition determines its appetite thereafter and hence its rate of growth and dimensions at maturity. A small size at this critical time brought about by undernutrition is not followed by catch-up growth, however liberal the diet.'

This concept of critical epochs in growth applies not only to the organism as a whole but to individual organs and most importantly to the brain. In fact, Dobbing and others (63) have shown that this sensitivity extends to individual cellular populations within the brain, developing on different time schedules, which can be selectively compromised by nutritional or other insult applied during a particular period of development. In the human premature, for example, glial proliferation and cerebellar development, general myelination and dendritic arborization (64) are still proceeding during the last trimester of intrauterine life and into the neonatal period. If an infant is born prematurely, the neonatologist has perforce to become the surrogate for the placenta, without unfortunately being endowed with all the subtle transfer and feedback mechanisms possessed by that remarkable organ. The neonatologist must ensure that these infants are provided with the means, not only to survive, but also to develop physically and mentally to their full genetic potential. An example which dramatizes the effect of undernutrition in one of two individuals with identical potentials is shown in Figure 16. These infants are parabiotic twins in whom the vascular arrangement of the placenta has deprived one of the pair. To what extent has this degree of malnutrition infringed on the 'sensitive period' of development? Is it not possible that we, as neonatal intensivists, may be witnessing a somewhat similar nutritional deprivation in some of the infants in our charge despite all our well-meant efforts? The infant may be too sick to absorb any nutrient from the gastrointestinal tract due to immaturity and/or ileus secondary to cardiorespiratory failure, infection or serious gastrointestinal or other anomaly. Such severe illness also compromises the ability of the organism adequately to metabolize intravenously administered nutrients, witness the frequent hyperglycemia, the early azotemia and inability to clear intravenously administered lipids. The immature or damaged liver is one of the key organs in this respect and is probably involved in the causation of the major macronutrient biochemical intolerance to carbohydr-

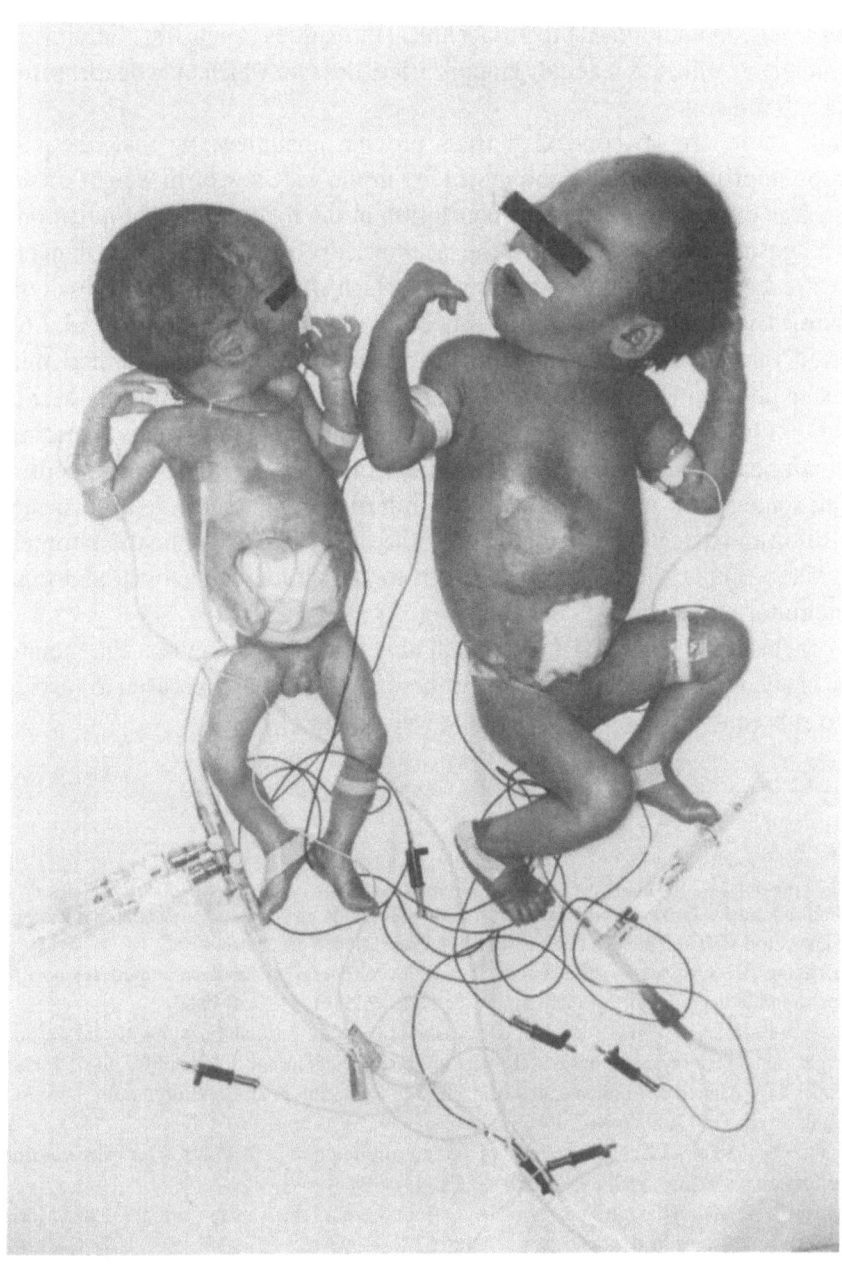

Figure 16. Monozygotic, parabiotic twins.

24

ate (hyperglycemia), lipids (hyperlipidemia), amino acids (abnormal serum levels for individual amino acids), raised BUN and other macro- and micronutrient serum levels. In addition, there are technical difficulties in substrate administration, defective utilization and/or inappropriate dosage, which may distort serum levels and utilization.

While there are no controlled trials proving unequivocally that adequate nutrition improves mortality and morbidity in the very low birth weight or sick infant, it is difficult to escape this conclusion in the light of modern nutritional knowledge and practice, despite the acknowledged difficulties and dangers. There are many other factors than nutrition which affect outcome of the high risk neonate. The observation period is necessarily prolonged. Stein et al. (65) reported that the underweight infant survivors of the sharply defined third trimester period of severe maternal starvation in Holland during the second World War in 1945, when examined at induction into the Army twenty years later could not be distinguished developmentally from their peers. Although controversial, some follow-up studies of growth-retarded infants show delay in speech acquisition and defects in developmental indices (66). There is animal experimental evidence implicating nutritional deprivation as a major factor in abnormal psychomotor and cognitive development (67).

In conclusion, I hope that I have been able to convince you that the maintenance of adequate nutrition in the sick or premature newborn is crucial to survival and to subsequent normal growth and development.

REFERENCES

1. Widdowson EM, Spray CM: Chemical development in utero. Arch Dis Child 26: 205–214, 1951
2. Widdowson EM: Growth and composition of the fetus and newborn. In Assali NS (ed), Biology of Gestation II. The Fetus and Neonate. Acad Press, New York, 1968
3. Reichman BL, Chessex P, Putet G et al.: Partition of energy metabolism and energy cost of growth in the very low birth weight infant. Pediatrics 69: (6), 446–451, 1982
4. Chessex P, Reichman BL, Verellen GJE et al.: Influence of postnatal age, energy intake and weight gain on energy metabolism in the very low birth weight infant. J Pediatr 99: 761–766, 1981
5. Scopes JW, Ahmed I: Minimal rates of oxygen consumption in sick and premature newborn infants. Arch Dis Child 66: 407, 1966
6. Bhakoo NN, Scopes JW: Minimal rates of oxygen consumption in small-for-dates babies during the first weeks of life. Arch Dis Childh 49: 583, 1974
7. Ashworth A: Metabolic rates during recovery from protein-calorie malnutrition: the need for a new concept of specific dynamic action. Nature 223: 407, 1969
8. Reid M, Reilly BJ, Murdock AI, Swyer PR: Cardiomegaly in association with neonatal hypoglycaemia. Acta Paed Scand 60: 295, 1971
9. Rowe RD, Izukawa T, Mulholland HC et al.: Non-structural heart disease in the newborn: observations during one year in a perinatal service. Arch Dis Child 53: 726, 1978
10. Heim T: Energy requirements of thermoregulatory heat production in the early born. In: Monset-Couchard M., Minkowski A. (eds), Physiological and Biochemical Basis for Perinatal Medicine. S. Karger, Basel, pp 158–174, 1981

11. Müller N, Gulston G, Cade D et al.: Diaphragmatic muscle fatigue in the newborn. J Appl Physiol: Respir Environ Exercise Physiol 46: 688, 1979

12. Budin PC: The Nursling. The feeding and hygiene of premature and full term infants. Authorized translation by WJ Maloney of 'Le Nourisson' (1900) Caxton Publishing Co, London, 1907

13. Bryan MH, Wei P, Hamilton JR et al.: Supplemental intravenous hyperalimentation in newborns less than 1300 grams. J Pediatr 82: 940, 1973

14. Holman RT: Essential fatty acid deficiency in humans. In Galli C, Jacini G, Pecile A (eds), Dietary Lipids and Postnatal Development. Raven Press, New York, p 127, 1973

15. Holman RT: Essential Fatty Acid Deficiency. Progress in Chemistry of Fat and Other Lipids. Pergamon Press, Inc New York, 279 pp, 1968

16. Holman RT: Essential fatty acid deficiency in humans. In Galli C, Jacini G, Pecile A (eds), Dietary Lipids and Postnatal Development. Raven Press, New York, p 127, 1973

17. Friedman Z, Danon MD, Stahlman MT, Oates JA: Rapid onset of essential fatty acid deficiency in the newborn. Pediatrics 58: 640, 1976

18. Shimoyana T, Kikuchi H, Press H, Thompson GR: Fatty acid composition of plasma lipoproteins in control subjects and in patients with malabsorption. Gut 14: 716, 1973

19. Thompson GR, Heath J, Press M: Changes in fatty acid composition of plasma lipoprotein during administration of intralipid to a patient with essential fatty acid deficiency. Clin Sci Mol Med 47: 387, 1974

20. Widdowson EM, Colombo VE, Artravius CA: Changes in the organs of pigs in response to feeding for the first 24 hours after birth. II. The digestive tract. Biol Neonate 28: 272–282, 1976

21. Widdowson EM: Gastrointestinal development and neonatal nutrition. Proceedings of the 72nd Ross Conference on Pediatric Research. Ross Laboratories, Columbus, Ohio, 1977

22. Pitcher-Wilmott R, Shutack JG, Fox WW: Decreased lung volume after nasogastric feeding of neonates recovering from respiratory disease. J Pediatr 95: 119–121, 1979

23. Brown EG, Sweet AY: Preventing necrotising enterocolitis in neonates. JAMA 240: 2452–2454, 1978

24. Roy RN, Pollnitz JR, Hamilton JR, Chance GW: Impaired assimilation of nasojejunal feeds in very low birth weight infants. J Pediatr 90: 431, 1977

25. Field T, Ignatieff E, Stringer S et al.: Nonnutritive sucking during tube feedings. Peditrics 70: 381, 1982

26. Batton DG, Maisels MJ, Appelbaum P: Peripheral intravenous catheters in premature infants: a controlled study. Pediatrics 70: 487–490, 1982

27. Broviac JW, Cole JJ, Scribner BH: A silicone rubber catheter for prolonged parenteral alimentation. Surg Gynecol Obstet 136: 602, 1973

28. Morgan WW, Heillen GW: Percutaneous introduction of long-term indwelling vascular catheters in infants. J Pediatr Surg 7: 538, 1972

29. Dolcourt JL, Bose CL: Percutaneous insertion of silastic central venous catheters in newborn infants. Pediatrics 70: 484–486, 1982

30. Widdowson EM, Spray M: Chemical development in utero. Arch Dis Child 26: 205–214, 1951

31. Widdowson EM: Growth and composition of the fetus and newborn. In: Assali NS (ed), Biology of Gestation II. The Fetus and Neonate. Acad Press, New York, 1968

32. Ziegler EE, O'Donnell AM, Nelson SE, Fomon SJ: Body composition of the reference fetus. Growth 40: 329–341, 1976

33. Atkinson SA, Anderson GH, Bryan MH: Human milk: comparison of the nitrogen composition of milk from mothers of premature and full term infants. Am J Clin Nutr 33: 811–815, 1980

34. Atkinson SA, Radde IC, Chance GW et al.: Macromineral content of milk obtained during early lactation from mothers of premature infants. Ear Hum Dev 4: 5–14, 1980

35. Chessex P, Reichman BL, Verellen GJE et al.: The quality of growth in premature infants fed own mothers' milk. J Pediatr 102: 107–112, 1983

36. Heird WC, Anderson TL: Nutritional requirements and methods of feeding low birth weight

26

infants. Curr Probl Pediatr 7: 3, 1977
37. Mead-Johnson, Nutritional Division: Enfamil Premature Formula Clinical Report. Evansville, Indiana, 1979
38. Ross Laboratories: Similac Special Care Infant Formula Product Handbook for the Growing Low Birth Weight Infant. Columbus, Ohio, 1980
39. Shenai JP, Reynolds JW, Babson SG: Nutritional balance studies in very low birth weight infants: enhanced nutrient retention rates by an experimental formula. Pediatrics 66: 233–238, 1980
40. Silverio J, Tomarelli R, Barness LA et al.: Results of feeding a special formula to very low birth weight (VLBW) infants. Presented to XVI International Congress of Pediatrics. Barcelona, Spain, September 1980
41. Wyeth Laboratories: Premie SMA Low Birth Weight Infant Formula Product Handbook. Philadelphia, 1981
42. Reichman BL, Chessex P, Verellen GJE et al.: Dietary composition and macronutrient storage in preterm infants. Pediatrics 72: 322, 1983
43. Reichman BL, Chessex P. Putet G et al.: Diet, fat accretion and growth in premature infants. New Engl J Med 305: 1495–1500, 1981
44. Anderson GH, Bryan MH (editorial): Is the premature infant's own mother's milk best? J Ped Gastroenterol Nutr 1: 157–159, 1982
45. Atkinson SA, Anderson GH, Bryan MH: Human milk: comparison of the nitrogen composition of milk from mothers of premature and full term infants. Am J Clin Nutr 33: 811–815, 1980
46. Chessex P, Reichman BL, Verellen GJE et al.: The quality of growth in premature infants few own mother's milk. J Pediatr 102: 107–112, 1983
47. Gordon HH, Levine SZ, McNamara H: Feeding of premature infant: comparison of human and cow's milks. Am J Dis Child 73: 442, 1947
48. Gross SJ, David RJ, Bauman L, Tomarelli RM: Nutritional composition of milk produced by mothers delivering preterm. J Pediatr 96: 641, 1980
49. Chance GW, Radde IC, Willis EM et al.: Postnatal growth of infants of less than 1.3 kg birth weight: effects of metabolic acidosis, calorie intake and of calcium, sodium and phosphate supplementation. J Pediatr 91: 787–793, 1977
50. Day GM, Chance GW, Radde IC et al.: Growth and mineral metabolism in very low birth weight infants: effects of calcium supplementation on growth and divalent cations. Pediatr Res 9: 568–574, 1975
51. Andrews BF, Lorch V: Improved fat and calcium absorption in low birth weight infants fed a medium-chain triglyceride containing formula. Pediatr Res 8: 104, 1974
52. Roy CC, Ste-Marie M, Chartrand L et al.: Correction of malabsorption of the preterm infant with medium-chain triglyceride formula. J Pediatr 86: 446, 1975
53. Tantibehedhyangkul P, Hashim SA: Medium-chain triglyceride feeding in premature infants: effects on fat and nitrogen absorption. Pediatrics 55: 359, 1975
54. Davd L, Anast CS: Calcium metabolism in newborn infants: the inter-relationship of parathyroid function and calcium, magnesium and phosphorus metabolism in normal, sick and hypocalcemic newborns. J Clin Invest 54: 287, 1974
55. David L, Salle BL, Putet G et al.: Serum immunoreactive calcitonin in low birth weight infants. Description of early changes: effect of intravenous calcium infusion; relationships with early changes in serum calcium, phosphorus, magnesium, parathyroid hormone and gastrin levels. Pediatr Res 15: 803, 1981
56. Filler RM, Takada Y, Carreras T, Heim T: Serum intralipid levels in neonates during parenteral nutrition: the relation to gestational age. J Pediatr Surg 15: 4, 1980
57. Forget PP, Fernandes J, Haverkampbegman P: Utilisation of fat emulsion during total parenteral nutrition. Acta Paed Scand 64: 377, 1975
58. Cross KW, Tizard JPM, Trythall DAH: The gaseous metabolism of the newborn infant. Acta Paed Scand 46: 265, 1957

59. Heim T, Putet G, Verellen GJE et al.: Energy cost of intravenous alimention in the newborn infant. In: Stern L, Salle B, Friis-Hansen B (eds), Intensive Care of the Newborn III. Masson Publishing New York, pp 219–238, 1981

60. Bryan MH, Shennan AT, Griffin E, Angel A: Intralipid - its rational use in parenteral nutrition of the newborn. Pediatrics 58: 787, 1976

61. Smigura FC, Bryan MH, Angel A: Postheparin lipase activity in newborn infants. In: Hahn P, Segal S, Israels S (eds), The Role of Fat in Intravenous Feeding of the Newborn. Pharmacia (Can) Ltd, Dorval, p 129, 1974

62. Widdowson EM, McCance RA: A review: New thoughts on growth. Pedatr Res 9: 154, 1975

63. Dobbing J: The later development of the central nervous system and its vulnerability. In: Davis JA, Dobbing J (eds), Scientific Foundations of Paediatrics. Saunders, Philadelphia, pp 565–577, 1974

64. Purpura DP: Dendritic differentiation in human cerebral cortex: normal and aberrant development patterns. In: Kreutzberg GW (ed), Physiology and Pathology of Dendrites (Advances in Neurology, Vol 12). Raven Press, New York, pp 91–116, 1975

65. Stein Z, Susser M, Saegner G, Morolla F: Famine and human development. The Dutch hunger winter of 1944–45. New York University Press, London, 1975

66. Davies PA, Stewart AL: Low birth weight infants: neurological sequels and later intelligence. Br Med Bull 31: 85–91, 1975

67. Canadian Paediatric Society Nutrition Committee: Feeding the low birth weight infant. Can Med Assoc J p 124, 1981

68. McGilvery RW: Storage of the major fuels. In: McGilvery RW (ed), Biochemistry, a Functional Approach, III. Saunders, Philadelphia, pp 287–459, 1970

69. Millward DG, Garlick PJ: The energy cost of growth. Proc Nutr Soc 35: 339–349, 1976

70. Heim T: Homeothermy and its metabolic cost. In: Davis JA, Dobbing J (eds), Medical Books Ltd, London, pp 91–128, 1981

71. Swyer PR: Crises and interventions in the nutrition of the high risk newborn. In: Shoemaker WC, Thompson WL (eds), Critical Care - State of the Art IV. Society for Critical Care Medicine, pp IV(M): 1 - IV(M):47, March, 1983

2. THE INDUCTION OF FETAL LUNG MATURATION

Ian Gross

INTRODUCTION

Respiratory distress syndrome of the newborn (RDS) is due to immaturity of the lungs at birth, particularly the surfactant system. The considerable mortality and morbidity associated with this condition has focused attention on the regulation of fetal lung development.

It is now generally accepted that the rate of fetal lung maturation is influenced by a number of circulating hormones (Table 1). Corticosteroids and thyroid hormones accelerate maturation, including surfactant synthesis, whereas beta-adrenergic agonists appear to stimulate surfactant secretion specifically (1). Epidermal growth factor also acts directly on the lung to enhance surfactant production and insulin and/or hyperglycemia may delay lung maturation, so that the final rate of this process may depend on interactions between a number of hormones. There is also some evidence that estrogens and prolactin enhance surfactant production, but the role of these agents is controversial at the present

Table 1. Hormones that influence fetal lung surfactant synthesis or secretion.

Enhancement
Corticosteroids
Thyroid hormones
Epidermal growth factor
Beta-adrenergic agonists
Inhibition
Insulin/hyperglycemia
? physiological role
Estrogen
Prolactin

time and it is not clear whether they play a physiological role in regulating fetal lung maturation.

In this review the multi-hormonal regulation of lung development and surfactant production will be discussed as well as a possible role for endogenous pulmonary factors in initiating this process.

MULTI-HORMONAL REGULATION OF LUNG DEVELOPMENT

Corticosteroids

The early studies by Liggins (2) and Avery and associates which demonstrated that fetal lung maturation could be accelerated by the administration of corticosteroids has led to a considerable amount of work in this area. It has now been shown that corticosteroids stimulate biochemical and physiological parameters of lung development as well as morphologic differentiation (1). These effects appear to occur concurrently. Specific receptors for glucocorticoids have been demonstrated in both fetal and adult lungs as well as in isolated alveolar type II cells (3). The current theory of corticosteroid action on the lung is that the hormone binds initially to specific receptors in the cytoplasm. The receptor–steroid complex is then translocated to the nucleus of the cell where new messenger RNA synthesis occurs. The messenger RNA sequences are ultimately translated into new protein synthesis in the cytoplasm so that enzymes of surfactant production or protein components of surfactant are then produced. Although there is considerable evidence that this mechanism does indeed operate in the lung, there is controversy as to which proteins are induced by corticosteroids. These hormones have been reported to increase the activity of phosphatidate phosphatase and cholinephosphate cytidylyltransferase, enzymes involved with phospholipid synthesis, although this finding has not held up in all studies (1). It is also not clear whether steroids induce new enzyme protein or merely activate these enzymes. What does appear to be clear, however, is that each hormone that acts on the lung acts at different sites initially and produces somewhat different effects (4).

There are good correlations between corticosteroid effects and corticosteroid binding (5). For example, the dose-response characteristics of binding and stimulation of phosphatidylcholine synthesis or cholinephosphate cytidylyltransferase activity are similar. (Dissaturated phosphatidylcholine is the major component of surfactant.) In addition, the potency of various steroids for the stimulation of phosphatidylcholine synthesis correlates well with the affinity of these steroids for the glucocorticoid receptor. Experimental evidence therefore supports the concept that corticosteroid effects are mediated by binding to specific receptors with subsequent synthesis of RNA and protein.

Corticosteroid action has not only been observed in animals. There are now a number of clinical trials in humans which have indicated that the incidence of RDS can be reduced by antenatal corticosteroid treatment (6,7). Since steroids act through new protein synthesis there is a time lag between administration of the hormone and the observation of their effect. For clinical effectiveness, a 24–48-hr interval between administration of hormone to the pregnant mother and delivery of the infant is necessary. In addition, it has been shown in both animals and man that steroid action is gestation-dependent. Corticosteroids act primarily on the immature lung; they are ineffective after about 34 weeks gestation in the human (6). The optimal time for steroid action appears to be between about 30 and 33 weeks. When steroids are used correctly (i.e. administered at an appropriate gestational age and only in those situations where at least 24 to 48 hr is likely to elapse between the time of administration of the drug and delivery of the infant), they have been shown in most studies to reduce the incidence of RDS by about 50–70%. Some recent studies have suggested that steroids may be less effective in males than in females (7).

Initial concerns regarding the use of corticosteroids focused primarily on possible detrimental effects of these hormones on brain development. Animal studies have shown that there is inhibition of cell multiplication in the cerebellum and cerebrum following corticosteroid treatment. Clinical studies, which have used much lower doses, have however not born this out. Follow-up studies from New Zealand where the largest clinical trial of corticosteroid administration was carried out have been favorable (8). With the advent of these developmental studies concerns have turned from the issue to toxicity to that of effectiveness. For this reason, the possibility of using combinations of hormones rather than one hormone alone to accelerate lung maturation is now under consideration. The question of hormone synergism will be discussed later in this chapter.

Epithelial–mesenchymal interactions

It has been known for some time that the development of the epithelial lining of the lung is dependent on the presence of mesenchymal tissue. Removal of all the mesenchymal tissue prevents development of the lung, but recombinations of epithelium and mesenchyme develop in a reasonably normal fashion (9). Corticosteroid action on the epithelial cells of the lung also appears to be dependent on the presence of mesenchymal tissue. Smith has shown that relatively pure populations of fetal human type II cells have a very small response to cortisol. If however, fibroblasts are exposed to cortisol and the resulting medium is collected and incubated with type II cells, there is considerable enhancement of surfactant synthesis. Smith has partially purified a factor known as the 'fibroblast pneumonocyte factor', which he believes is synthesized by fibroblasts in response to corticosteroids (10). The hypothesis is that corticosteroid action on fibroblasts results in the production of this factor which in turn acts on the type II cells, probably via a membrane receptor and cyclic AMP-mediated mechanism. Injection of the factor into rats in vivo has been shown to promote biochemical maturation of the lung. It is possible that corticosteroids act directly on epithelial cells and also via the mesenchymal cells and the combination of these two effects results in accelerated lung maturation.

Thyroid hormone

A number of thyroid hormones and thyroid hormone analogues have been shown to stimulate lung maturation (11). Triodothyronine (T_3) appears to be among the most potent of these agents. Specific nuclear receptors for thyroid hormones have been demonstrated in fetal lung (12) and as is the case with corticosteroids, the potency of various thyroid analogues for stimulating surfactant production appears to correlate with the affinity for binding.

Although they accelerate lung maturation and surfactant production, thyroid hormones do not produce the same effects as do corticosteroids. For example, whereas corticosteroids increase the relative synthesis of disaturated phosphatidylcholine and phosphatidylglycerol in organ cultures of fetal rat lung, thyroid hormones do not (4). They appear to work through different mechanisms than the corticosteroids.

Thyroid hormones (T_3 and T_4) in general do not cross the placenta freely and studies of their effects in vivo have been hindered by the fact that the hormones must be injected directly into fetuses. This procedure in and of itself can stimulate lung maturation. Interest has therefore been centered on thyrotropin-releasing hormone (TRH), a tripeptide which crosses the placenta readily in most species studied. Administration of this agent to pregnant rabbits stimulates lung maturation, and it has been suggested that it may be useful clinically (13). There have been no large clinical studies of the effectiveness of thyroid hormones in preventing RDS, but small studies which were not controlled have suggested that intra-amniotic administration of T_4 may reduce the incidence of RDS (14). Concerns relating to the intra-amniotic injection hormone have delayed clinical use of those hormones.

Thyroid hormones also augment the effects of corticosteroids on lung maturation and recent interest in these hormones has tended to focus on their additive or synergistic interactions with the corticosteroids.

Insulin

Fetuses of diabetic mothers have both increased insulin and glucose levels. Glucose crosses the placenta freely from the hyperglycemic mother to the fetus and stimulates insulin production by the fetal pancreas. Insulin does not cross the placenta freely. These infants have an increased incidence of RDS compared to gestationally matched infants from nondiabetic pregnancies (15). This clinical observation has led to a number of experimental studies, but at present the precise reason for the delayed lung maturation is not clear. Part of the problem is that it has been difficult to establish appropriate animal models. Whereas the human infants of diabetic mothers are generally large for gestational age and hyperinsulinemic, many of the animal models have resulted in fetuses that are normal or small in weight and normoinsulinemic. In some animal studies delayed lung maturation has been demonstrated and in others this has not been the case.

Attempts to study insulin action on the lung in vitro have also produced conflicting results. Studies from our laboratory and others have shown that insulin delays various parameters of lung maturation including morphologic development and decreases the synthesis of the surfactant phospholipids (16). It appears that insulin may antagonize the action of glucocorticoids so that the stimulatory effect of these steroids on lung maturation in tissue culture is abolished by the addition of insulin to the culture medium (17). Other studies however have not shown delayed lung maturation. Because the animal models are sometimes hyperglycemic but normoinsulinemic, there has been speculation that it may be the hyperglycemia and not the hyperinsulinemia which causes the delayed lung maturation. Whatever the mechanism, it is clear that in diabetic pregnancies that are not tightly controlled the infants are large and have an increased incidence of RDS. If the pregnancy is tightly controlled and the infants are allowed to go to term, the incidence of RDS is not higher than in normal infants.

It is of interest that lungs which have been exposed to insulin contain large amounts of glycogen. Glycogen is thought to be a precursor for lung phospholipid synthesis and it is possible that there is failure of glycogen degradation in the infants resulting in decreased surfactant production (16). Conversely, those agents which are known to stimulate surfactant production such as corticosteroids, thyroid hormones, and cyclic AMP produce an increase in glycogen breakdown (1). This inverse relationship between glycogen content and surfactant production is also seen during normal development (18), further supporting the view that glycogen breakdown is in some way linked with the onset of surfactant phospholipid synthesis.

Beta-adrenergic agonists

A number of studies have shown that beta-adrenergic agonists such as epinephrine increase the secretion of the surfactant phospholipids. It is not clear whether they increase synthesis as well. The effect of these agents is however observed within a few hours of exposure, consistent with an effect on secretion rather than synthesis. The beta-agonists appear to act directly on the alveolar epithelial cells and a number of studies have demonstrated increased secretion of surfactant phospholipids in isolated adult type II cells after exposure to these agents (19). It is believed that the beta-agonists bind to receptors on the membrane of the type II cell with activation of the adenylate cyclase mechanism and production of cyclic AMP. Specific receptors have been demonstrated in both fetal and adult lung. During fetal development the concentration of beta-adrenergic receptors on the surface of the lung cells increases. This increase is enhanced by corticosteroids (20) and thyroxine (21). Thus one of the ways in which these hormones influence lung maturation may be by increasing the ability of the type II cells to secrete surfactant as a consequence of increased beta-adrenergic binding capacity.

The role of cholinergic agents in surfactant synthesis is less clear. It has been shown that these agents stimulate surfactant secretion in vivo (22) but not in vitro. This suggests that their action on the type II cell is an indirect one. For example cholinergic agents may increase epinephrine production by the adrenal with resulting enhancement of surfactant secretion.

Estrogen

The physiological role of estrogen in lung maturation is not clear. In most species there is a considerable increase in estrogen levels towards the end of gestation and it has been shown in the rabbit that administration of estrogen to the mother results in significant enhancement of fetal lung surfactant production (23). In organ culture, however, high levels of this steroid were required to produce an increase in surfactant phospholipid synthesis (24). Thus the direct effects of estrogen in vitro were not noted at physiological levels. Receptors for estrogen have been described in both human (25) and fetal rabbit lung, but they appear to differ from the classical estrogen receptor in their binding properties, again casting doubt on the physiological role of estrogen.

Prolactin

In both humans and sheep the rise in fetal plasma prolactin levels precedes the increase in surfactant production. This has led to speculation that prolactin may be important for initiating fetal lung maturation (26). In addition, injection of prolactin to fetal rabbits was reported to be associated with a marked increase in lung tissue disaturated phosphatidylcholine content (27). However, other studies have failed to confirm this finding and prolactin was reported to have no effect on surfactant production in fetal sheep (28). Tissue culture experiments have produced conflicting results. At present the role of prolactin in fetal lung maturation is ill defined and the subject of some controversy.

Hormone synergism

The recent collaborative study of dexamethasone administration for the prevention of RDS (7) suggested that glucocorticoids might not be as effective for this purpose as was previously believed. Attention is now turning to more potent ways of stimulating lung maturation in the fetus and one of these might be the administration of hormone combinations rather than single hormones. In a number of organs other than the lung, there are synergistic interactions between T_3 and glucocorticoids. We have shown in explants of fetal rat lung that there are additive interactions between T_3 and glucocorticoids with regard to phospholipid synthesis (29) and this observation has also now been noted with fetal rabbit lung. Smith and Sabry (30) have reported that T_3 sensitizes fetal type II cells to the action of the 'fibroblast pneumonocyte factor' which is produced by fibroblasts after exposure to glucocorticoids.

Since there was considerable in vitro evidence that interactions between glucocorticoids and T_3 occurred in fetal lung, we also undertook a study of these interactions in vivo in the rat (31). T_3 was injected directly into the mother in large amounts and by measuring fetal serum T_3 levels we demonstrated that there was significant passage of this hormone across the placenta. (In most species there is very little passage of thyroid hormones from mother to fetus.) As was the case in vitro, additive effects of betamethasone and T_3 on surfactant phospholipid synthesis were demonstrated in the fetuses after maternal injection of these hormones suggesting that combined hormone administration may also be effective for clinical purposes. Although thyroid hormones do not cross the human placenta to any significant extent, some thyroid analogues and thyrotropin-releasing hormone (TRH) do. We had shown earlier that TRH stimulates some parameters of surfactant production in the fetal rabbit (11) and this raises the possibility that TRH may be useful clinically for preventing RDS particularly when used in combination with corticosteroids. Controlled clinical trials of combined hormone administration would appear to be a real possibility in the not too distant future.

The initiation of fetal lung maturation

Although fetal lung maturation is influenced by a number of hormones it has not been established that circulating hormones are responsible for initiating this process. Since the levels of a number of hormones including corticosteroids and prolactin increase during the last trimester of gestation, there has been speculation in the literature that the rise in the levels of these hormones may initiate the production of pulmonary surfactant. Although corticosteroids almost certainly play a role in the physiological regulation of fetal lung maturation and thyroid hormones have been shown to accelerate lung development in a number of species, it is not clear that any of these agents initiate this process. The fact that there are temporal associations between rising hormone levels and surfactant production does not necessarily mean that there is a causal relationship between these events.

We examined the maturation of explants of fetal rat lung of 13–20 days gestation in a culture system where there could be no surge in hormone levels (32). Irrespective of the gestational age of the lungs used, there was a marked increase in surfactant phospholipid synthesis at approximately the same time as would have occurred in vivo. (The normal increase starts at day 18 and then accelerates markedly at day 20 in the rat. In culture there was a similar increase at an equivalent gestational age of 18 days, i.e. 13 day lungs after 5 days in culture, or 16 day lungs after 2 days in culture.) Other parameters of lung maturation also continued in the absence of a surge in hormone levels. There was evidence of continuing morphologic development, an increase in the DNA content of the cultures, and an increase in the glucocorticoid binding capacity which closely paralleled the increase which normally occurs in vivo. The fact that these four parameters of lung development increased in this culture system strongly suggests that the stimulus for the initiation of fetal lung maturation is located in the lung tissue itself. Removal of up to 75% of the mesenchymal tissue did not delay lung maturation. This could be interpreted as implying either that small amounts of mesenchymal tissue are adequate for this process or that the message for the initiation of lung maturation is contained within the epithelial cells. Our findings therefore suggest that circulating hormones do not initiate the maturation of the fetal rat lung. Their role is rather later modulation and enhancement of this process.

CONCLUSIONS

Fetal lung development is under multi-hormonal control. These hormones interact with each other with synergistic or antagonistic effects. The overall rate of lung maturation may ultimately depend on the combined effect of these various hormones. Although hormones regulate the rate of lung maturation it is not clear that they initiate this process. This appears to be determined by factors within the lung tissue itself. Recent animal studies suggest that corticosteroids and thyroid hormones have additive effects on lung maturation both in vivo and in vitro. It is possible that administration of combinations of hormones may prove to be more effective in preventing RDS in humans than administration of single hormones.

ACKNOWLEDGEMENTS

This work was supported by National Institutes of Health Grant HL 19752. Much of the work was done in collaboration with Dr Seamus A. Rooney and with the assistance of Christine M. Wilson and Diane W. Dynia.

REFERENCES

1. Gross I: The hormonal regulation of fetal lung maturation. Clin Perinatol 6:377–395, 1979
2. Liggens GC: Premature delivery of foetal lambs infused with glucocorticoids. J Endocrinol 45:515–523, 1969
3. Ballard PL, Mason RJ, Douglas WHJ: Glucocorticoid binding by isolated lung cells. Endocrinology 102:1570–1575, 1978
4. Gross I, Wilson CM, Ingleson LD, Brehier A, Rooney SA: Fetal lung in organ culture. III. Comparison of dexamethasone, thyroxine and methylxanthines. J Appl Physiol 48:872–877, 1980
5. Gross I, Ballard PL, Ballard RA, Jones CT, Wilson CM: Corticosteroid stimulation of phosphatidylcholine synthesis in cultured fetal rabbit lung. Evidence for de novo protein synthesis mediated by glucocorticoid receptors. Endocrinoloy 112:829–837, 1983
6. Liggens GC, Howie RN: A controlled trial of antepartum glucocorticoid treatment for prevention of respiratory distress syndrome in premature infants. Pediatrics 50:515–524, 1972
7. Collaborative group on antenatal steroid therapy: Effect of antenatal dexamethasone administration on the prevention of respiratory distress syndrome. Am J Obstet Gynecol 141:276–286, 1981
8. MacArthur BA, Howie RN, Dezoete JA, Elkins J: School progress and cognitive development of 6-year old children whose mothers were treated antenatally with betamethasone. Pediatrics 70:99–105, 1982
9. Masters JR: Epithelial mesenchymal interaction during lung development: the effect of mesenchymal mass. Devel Biol 51:98–108, 1976
10. Smith BT: Lung maturation in the fetal rat: acceleration by injection of fibroblast-pneumonocyte factor. Science 204:1094–1095, 1979
11. Ballard PL, Benson BJ, Brehier A, Carter JP, Kriz BM, Jorgensen EL: Transplacental stimulation of lung development in the fetal rabbit by 3,5-dimethyl-3'isopropyl-L-thyronine. J Clin Invest 65:1407–1417, 1980
12. Lindenberg JA, Brehier A, Ballard PL: Triodothyronine nuclear binding in fetal and adult rabbit lung and cultured lung cells. Endocrinology 103:1725–1731, 1978
13. Rooney SA, Marino PA, Gobran LI, Gross I, Warshaw JB: Thyrotropin-releasing hormone increases the amount of surfactant in lung lavage from fetal rabbits. Pediatr Res 13:623–625, 1979
14. Mashiach S, Barkai G, Sack J, Stern E, Goldman B, Brish M, Serr DM: Enhancement of fetal lung maturity by intra-amniotic administration of thyroid hormone. Am J Obstet Gynecol 130:289–293, 1978
15. Robert MF, Neff RK, Hubbell JP, Taeusch HW, Avery ME: Association between maternal diabetes and the respiratory-distress syndrome in the newborn. N Engl J Med 294:357–360, 1976
16. Gross I, Smith GJW, Wilson CM, Maniscalco WM, Ingleson LD, Brehier A, Rooney SA: The influence of hormones on the biochemical development of fetal rat lung in organ culture. II. Insulin. Pediatr Res 14:834–838, 1980
17. Smith BT, Giroud CJP, Robert M, Avery ME: Insulin antagonism of cortisol action on lecithin synthesis by cultured fetal lung cells. J Pediatr 87:953–955, 1975
18. Maniscalco WM, Wilson CM, Gross I, Gobran L, Rooney SA, Warshaw JB: Development of glycogen and phospholipid metabolism in fetal and newborn rat lung. Biochim Biophys Acta 530:333–346, 1978
19. Dobbs LG, Mason RJ: Pulmonary alveolar type II cells isolated from rats. Release of phosphatidylcholine in response to β-adrenergic stimulation. J Clin Invest 63:378–387, 1979
20. Cheng JB, Goldfien A, Ballard PL, Roberts JM: Glucocorticoids increase pulmonary β-adre-

nergic receptors in fetal rabbit. Endocrinology 107:1646–1648, 1980

21. Whitsett JA, Darovec-Beckerman C, Adams K, Pollinger J, Needleman H: Thyroid dependent maturation of β-adrenergic receptors in the rat lung. Biochem Biophys Res Commun 97:913–917, 1980

22. Corbet AJS, Flax P, Rudolph AJ: Reduced surface tension in lungs of fetal rabbits injected with pilocarpine. J Appl Physiol 41:7–14, 1976

23. Khosla SS, Rooney SA: Stimulation of fetal lung surfactant production by administration of 17 β-estradiol to the maternal rabbit. Am J Obstet Gynecol 133:213–216, 1979

24. Gross I, Wilson CM, Ingleson LD, Brehier A, Rooney SA: The influence of hormones on the biochemical development of fetal rat lung in organ culture. I.Estrogen.Biochim Biophys Acta 575:375–383, 1980

25. Mendelson CR, MacDonald PC, Johnston JM: Estrogen binding in human fetal lung tissue cytosol. Endocrinology 106:368–374, 1980

26. Hauth JC, Parker CR, MacDonald PC, Porter JC, Johnston JM: A role of fetal prolactin in lung maturation. Obstet Gynecol 51:81–88, 1978

27. Hamosh M, Hamosh P: The effect of prolactin on the lecithin content of fetal rabbit lung. J Clin Invest 59:1002–1005, 1977

28. Ballard PL, Gluckman PD, Brehier A, Kitterman JA, Kaplan SL, Rudolph AM, Grumbach MM: Failure to detect an effect of prolactin on pulmonary surfactant and adrenosteroids in fetal sheep and rabbits. J Clin Invest 62:879–883, 1978

29. Gross I, Wilson CM: Fetal lung in organ culture. IV. Supra additive hormone interactions. J Appl Physiol 52:1420–1425, 1982

30. Smith BT, Sabry K: Glucocorticoid-thyroid synergism in lung maturation: mechanism involving epithelial-mesenchymal interaction. Proc Natl Acad Sci USA 80:1951–1954, 1982

31. Gross I, Dynia DW, Wilson CM, Ingleson LD, Gewolb IH, Rooney SA: Glucocorticoid-thyroid hormone interactions in fetal rat lung. Pediatr Res 18:191–196, 1984

32. Gross I, Wilson CM: Fetal lung maturation. Initiation and modulation. J Appl Physiol 55:1725–1732, 1983

3. CEREBRAL BLOOD FLOW

M. Douglas Jones Jr.

INTRODUCTION

Measurement of cerebral blood flow (CBF) in the animal laboratory and on the clinical service differs in methodology and to a certain extent in rationale. This review will include a brief discussion of experiments from our own laboratory that compare the regulation of CBF in fetal, newborn and adult animals, followed by a comment on the advantages and shortcomings of CBF measurements on the clinical service. I will attempt to put CBF measurements in some perspective. The principal disadvantage of measuring CBF alone, in either the laboratory or clinical situation, is that CBF is just one of a number of variables that determine the brain's well-being. A CBF value has to be considered in the context of cerebral energy requirements, on the one hand, and blood metabolic substrate concentrations on the other. The real criterion of the adequacy of CBF in an hypoxic subject, for example, is the functional state of the brain. New techniques of neurological monitoring that promise to give the clinician direct access to the brain's level of function and its metabolic energy status will be mentioned at the end of the review.

THE CEREBRAL VASCULAR BED IN FETAL, NEWBORN AND ADULT SHEEP

Hypoxic hypoxia

In the face of an hypoxic stress, cerebral oxygen consumption ($CMRO_2$) can be maintained in one of two ways. CBF can increase enough to maintain oxygen delivery (OD) to the brain. Used in this sense OD is the product of CBF and the arterial oxygen content (the total amount of oxygen per ml of arterial blood). Alternatively, the brain can extract a larger fraction of the OD, minimizing the need for an increase in CBF. In that case OD would fall along with the arterial oxygen content, and the ratio $CMRO_2/OD$, i.e. the cerebral fractional oxygen extraction (E), would rise.

An example of these alternatives can be found in skeletal muscle (1, 2). Muscle at rest has a low fractional oxygen extraction; muscle oxygen delivery is relatively high. Hypoxic hypoxia (low PO_2) causes little increase in flow; instead the fractional oxygen extraction increases. Exercising muscle, in contrast, has a higher initial fractional extraction and relies on an increase in blood flow to maintain oxygen delivery, thus minimizing any further rise in fractional oxygen extraction. Either approach has its limitations. In an effort to maintain OD, the CBF can increase only so much. This is especially obvious in species in which the brain already receives a large proportion of cardiac output (3). On the other hand, an increase in E will eventually decrease the capillary PO_2 to a level incompatible with tissue oxygen uptake (1, 4).

Acute isocapnic (constant PCO_2) hypoxia hypoxia severe enough to lower arterial oxygen content by 50–75% is not associated with a change in $CMRO_2$. This applies equally well to fetal (5), newborn (<14 days) (6) and adult (7) sheep. However, the mechanism by which $CMRO_2$ is maintained differs among the three. In adults, OD is very well maintained and E does not change (Figure 1) (8). This is consistent with data from adults of other species (6). In the fetus and lamb, E rises somewhat (Figure 1) because OD is not as well maintained.

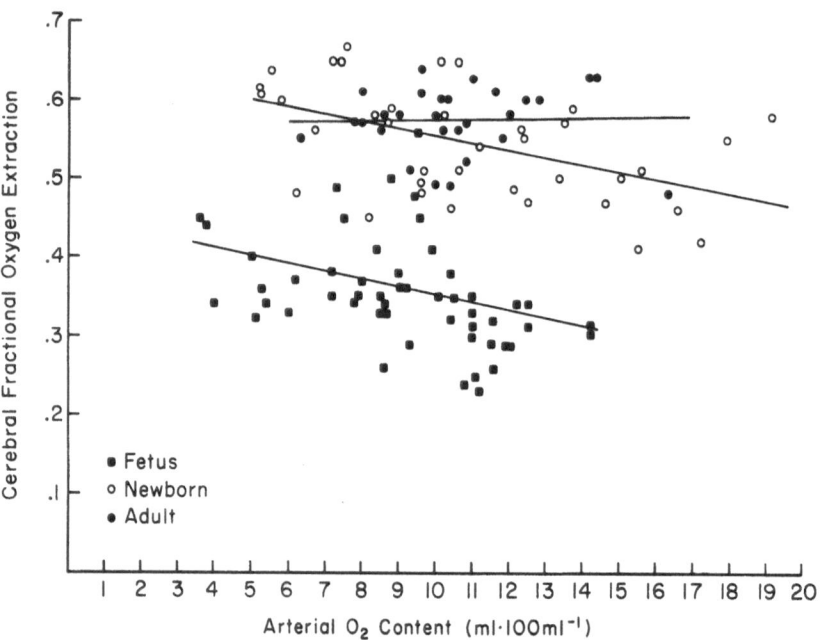

Figure 1. Cerebral fractional oxygen extraction in fetal, newborn and adult sheep during acute isocapnic hypoxic hypoxia. Both fetal and newborn regressions are significant ($p<0.01$). Reproduced with permission from Jones et al. (8).

By analogy to muscle, the more precise control of OD in the adult may relate to a higher baseline E value. E is 0.50–0.60 in the adult while in the fetus it is 0.25–0.35 (8). Results in the lamb are intermediate in the sense that in one study, E tended to rise (6) while in another, it was well maintained (9).

The low baseline fetal value of E is not uniquely characteristic of immaturity or of intrauterine existence. It appears to be primarily a function of the high oxygen affinity of fetal hemoglobin (10).

If one hypothesizes that CBF is controlled according to a tissue PO_2 level (11, 12), it follows that as oxyhemoglobin affinity rises and thus P_{50} (the PO_2 associated with 50% hemoglobin saturation) decreases, CBF will increase. The reasoning would be that as P_{50} falls, the capillary PO_2 for any arterial oxygen content will fall (Figure 2), and CBF at any oxygen content will increase. As a result, OD, which is the product of CBF and arterial oxygen content, will be higher.

This hypothesis is supported by data in both fetal sheep (10) and lambs (13). The P_{50} in adult sheep blood is 40 Torr and the P_{50} in the fetal sheep is 20 Torr. The

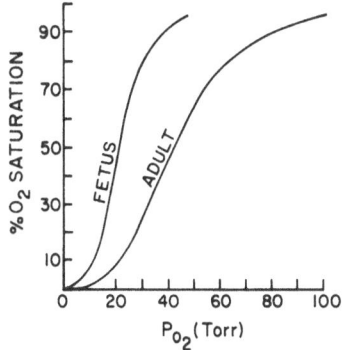

Figure 2. Fetal and adult (type B hemogoblin) oxyhemoglobin dissociation curves in sheep.

P_{50} in lamb blood is intermediate between 20 and 40 Torr as a result of the postnatal rise in 2,3 DPG (14) and the replacement of fetal hemoglobin synthesis by adult (15). If either the fetal sheep (10) or the lamb (13) is exchange transfused with adult sheep blood, OD falls and E rises toward adult levels (Figure 3). The hypothesis is also supported by increased CBF in adult man with a high-affinity hemoglobin variant (16).

Whether the fetus or lamb will be precise in maintaining the higher postexchange transfusion value of E is an important unanswered question. It is not clear why E rises in hypoxic fetuses before exchange transfusion (8). The rise in E might represent a somewhat passive response in a relatively over-perfused organ, a direct analogy to resting muscle.

The rise in E does not represent an inability of fetal CBF to increase. Several

42

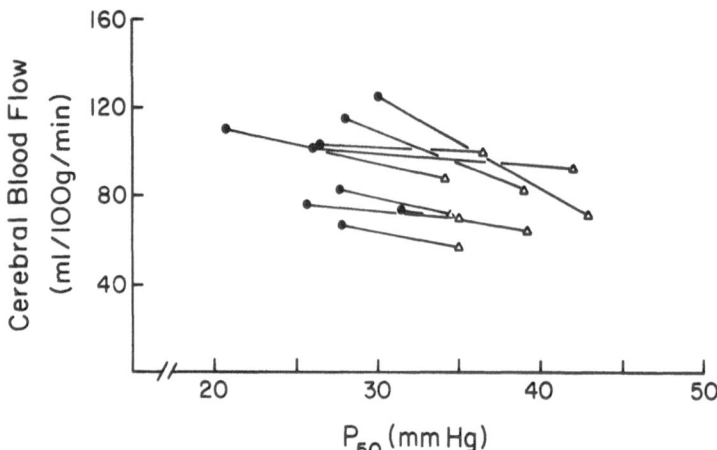

Figure 3. Cerebral fractional oxygen extraction in lambs before (●) and after (△) exchange transfusion with adult sheep red cells.

studies show that fetal CBF can increase considerably (17, 18) (Figure 4). Finally, it is possible that fetal (and newborn lamb) cerebral vessels are somewhat less sensitive to hypoxia, either as a primary phenomenon or secondary to circulating or endogenous vasodilators. Levels of the latter might increase in response to the stress of surgery in the fetus. It is evident that more studies are required.

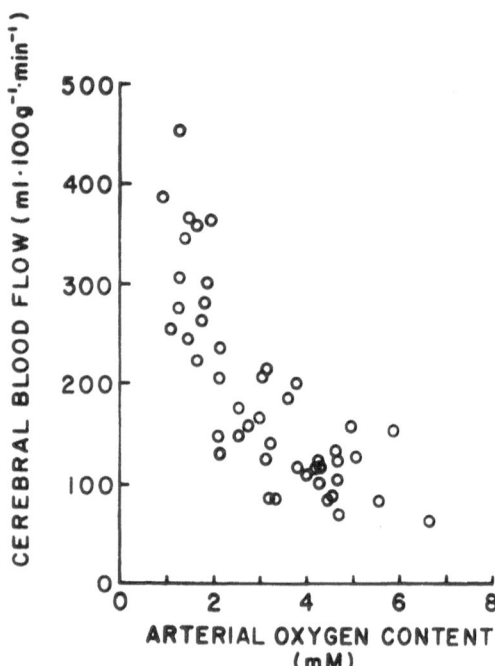

Figure 4. Cerebral blood flow in the fetal sheep as arterial oxygen content falls with acute isocapnic hypoxic hypoxia.

Anemic hypoxia

Results in anemic hypoxia are similar to those in hypoxic hypoxia, with the caveat that anemia has not been as well studied. In adults, $CMRO_2$ is maintained in acute isovolemic anemia (18), and in studies in which it can be calculated, E is not substantially changed (6, 18). In lambs a fall in hematocrit from 40 to 20% does not change $CMRO_2$ or E (6). In fetal sheep only OD has been measured. Preliminary data (19) suggest that OD tends to be maintained in acute anemia, but the data are insufficient to rule out a modest fall.

Carbon monoxide hypoxia

Carbon monoxide (CO) hypoxia differs from hypoxic and anemic hypoxia in two ways: the CBF response in adult sheep (7), adult humans (21) and lambs (9) is larger; and $CMRO_2$ falls, at least in adult sheep (7) and goats (22). As a result, E falls sharply in CO hypoxia (Figure 5).

The difference in CBF response correlates with the decrease in P_{50} that occurs when CO combines with hemoglobin (23). As CO occupies oxygen binding sites on the hemoglobin molecule, the oxygen affinity of the remaining sites increases (Figure 6).

It is not immediately clear how a shift in the dissociation curve explains the brisker CBF response with CO hypoxia. After all, capillary PO_2 falls in hypoxic hypoxia as well; indeed cerebral venous PO_2 is no different in CO and hypoxic hypoxia (9, 24) (Figure 7). Nevertheless, the fall in E in lambs with CO hypoxia is

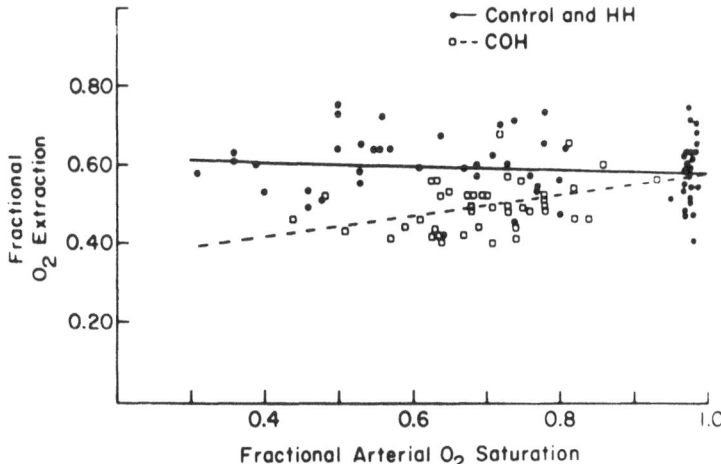

Figure 5. Cerebral fractional oxygen extraction as fractional arterial O_2 saturation falls in acute isocapnic hypoxic hypoxia and CO hypoxia in lambs. Reproduced with permission from Koehler et al. (9).

44

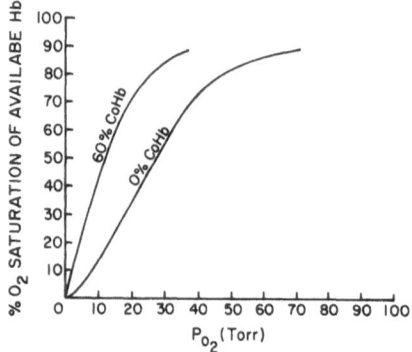

Figure 6. Changes in oxygen affinity of hemoglobin with increase in carboxyhemoglobin (COHb) saturation.

exactly that to be expected from the shift in the oxyhemoglobin dissociation curve (13). If lambs are first exchange transfused with adult blood, raising the P_{50} and increasing E, and then subsequently exposed to CO so that the P_{50} falls back to the control level, E also falls back to the control value.

The fall in $CMRO_2$ in adult sheep and goats is unexplained, but it may represent a direct effect of CO on cytochrome oxidase. CO, like cyanide, can combine with cytochrome a_3 (25). In normally oxygenated tissue, binding is minimal, but as tissue PO_2 falls, it could theoretically be enough to interfere with electron transport and therefore oxygen uptake (26). Alternatively, CO might reduce cytochrome oxidase activity indirectly, by diminishing mitochrondrial number (27).

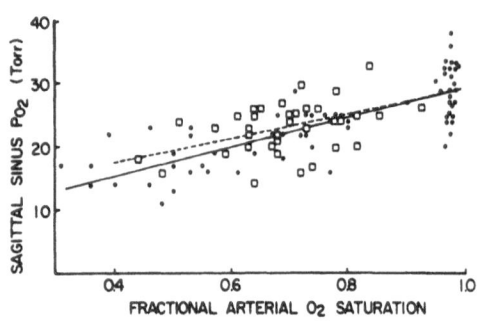

Figure 7. Cerebral venous (superior sagittal sinus) PO_2 in lambs as fractional arterial O_2 saturation falls with hypoxic hypoxia (●) and CO hypoxia (□). Reproduced with permission from Koehler et al. (9).

Hypercapnia

Among adult subjects with various types of CNS pathology, there is a close correlation between $CMRO_2$ and CO_2 responsiveness (28). Extrapolating from this observation, Hernandez et al. (29) speculated that the generally less vigorous CBF response to CO_2 in immature animals can be attributed to their lower $CMRO_2$. However, although differences in $CMRO_2$ correlate with developmental differences in CO_2 responsiveness in dogs (29) and Rhesus monkeys (30), a study of the fetal, newborn and adult sheep (31) shows that differences persist even after correction for $CMRO_2$ (Figure 8). In the sheep, $CMRO_2$ in the fetus is virtually the same as the adult; in the lamb it is higher than in the adult (31). Yet the correlation between immaturity and a lower CO_2 response persists: even after correction for $CMRO_2$, CO_2 responsiveness is significantly greater in the adult than in either fetus or lamb. Intrinsic differences among fetus, lamb and adult must therefore be important. The mechanism that links changes in PCO_2 to changes in CBF in adults is thought to be changes in the perivascular pH (32). This mechanism has not been demonstrated in immature animals, but it is unlikely to differ. Lesser CO_2 responsiveness might represent changes in the

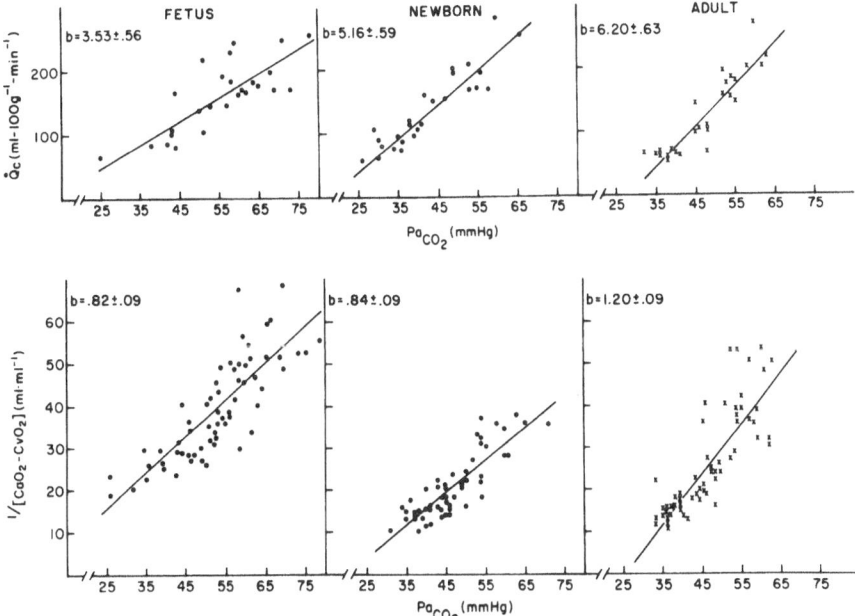

Figure 8. Upper panels show cerebral blood flow ($\dot{Q}_c$) in fetal sheep (130 days of gestation), lambs (<10 days of age) and adult sheep with acute hypercapnia. Fetal–adult differences are significant ($p<0.05$). Lower panels show $CBF/CMRO_2$ ($1/(CaO_2-CvO_2)$) in same experimental subjects. Fetal–adult and newborn–adult differences are significant ($p<0.05$). Regression coefficients (b) are mean ±SEM. Adult response is significantly greater than fetus or newborn even after correction for $CMRO_2$. Reproduced with permission from Rosenberg et al. (31).

sensitivity of individual vessels or it might be simply the result of a lower cerebrovascular density in the fetus and lamb.

CEREBRAL BLOOD FLOW MEASUREMENT IN THE INTENSIVE CARE UNIT

Measurement of CBF in humans began with the studies of Kety and Schmidt in 1945 (33). Over the next ten years investigators used this technique and its modifications to establish the basic principles of cerebrovascular physiology (34).

The purposes of CBF measurements on the modern clinical service are different (see Ref. 35). Techniques that map regional CBF are extraordinarily useful tools to identify such abnormalities as seizure foci, neoplasms and areas of circulatory compromise (35). CBF has also been measured in the intensive care unit, but here its usefulness is not so evident. In a patient with posttraumatic or postischemic cerebral edema, the clinician needs to decide when CBF has fallen to a critical level requiring mannitol infusion or surgical decompression or when CBF hyperemia is contributing to increased intracranial pressure. It is not clear that a CBF value is a more useful criterion for intervention in the individual patient than cerebral perfusion pressure and the neurological examination. One would also hope that CBF levels could predict outcome in patients with CNS damage. But aside from patients with either extremely low or very high blood flow CBF measurements are not necessarily indicative (35, 36). Complicating the issue enormously is the lack of a normal range for a particular brain region and clinical situation. One missing variable is regional metabolic rate. For example, pentobarbital coma lowers both $CMRO_2$ and CBF in equivalent fashion (37). It would therefore make no physiological sense to keep CBF in such an individual within the 'normal range'. But the situation is unfortunately rarely so clear as in pentobarbital coma. The interaction of cerebral pathology with anesthetic agents and other drugs (38) can have unpredictable effects on CBF, and even on the relationship between CBF and $CMRO_2$ (35).

A way out of this dilemma may be forthcoming from techniques like metabolic nuclear magnetic resonance (NMR) (39) and cortical-evoked potentials (40). Metabolic NMR permits noninvasive quantitation of high-energy phosphate concentrations in living tissue. This gives a picture of the relationship between cerebral oxygen delivery and cerebral oxygen consumption, a biochemical equivalent, if you will, of E. It clearly represents a step beyond the measurement of CBF alone. At present, metabolic NMR is applicable only to a somewhat indefinite region of the brain just under a 'surface coil' placed on the scalp. But it is not inconceivable that technical advances will achieve 3-dimensional tomographic mapping tissue of phosphate concentrations.

Evoked potentials assess CNS function directly. They can be obtained repeatedly over a short enough period of time to be helpful in the intensive care unit or even in the operating room (40).

SUMMARY

Work in experimental animals shows that the response of CBF to changes in the respiratory gases operate according to principles that are the same in the fetus as they are after birth. Subtle differences between fetus and adult do not contradict this general statement. Ironically, a more thorough understanding of the physiology of CBF has made it clear that CBF alone will be a variable of limited usefulness in the intensive care unit. Newer techniques, like cortical-evoked potentials and metabolic NMR, hold great promise if they prove practical in common clinical situations.

REFERENCES

1. Granger HJ, Goodman AH, Cook BH: Metabolic models of microcirculatory regulation. Fed Proc 34:2025–2030, 1975
2. Granger HJ, Goodman AH, Granger DN: Role of resistance and exchange vessels in local microvascular control of skeletal muscle oxygenation in the dog. Circ Res 38:379–385, 1976
3. Behrman RE, Lees MH: Organ blood flows of the fetal, newborn and adult rhesus monkey. Biol Neonate 18:330–340, 1971
4. Kreuzer F: Oxygen supply to tissues: the Krogh model and its assumptions. Experientia 38:1415–1426, 1982
5. Jones MD Jr, Sheldon RE, Peeters LL, Meschia G, Battaglia FC, Makowski EL: Fetal cerebral oxygen consumption at different levels of oxygenation. J Appl Physiol 43:1080–1084, 1977
6. Jones MD Jr, Traystman RJ, Simmons MA, Molteni RA: Effects of changes in arterial O_2 content on cerebral blood flow in the lamb. Am J Physiol 240 (Heart Circ Physiol 9):H209–H215, 1981
7. Koehler RC, Traystman RJ, Zeger S, Rogers MC, Jones MD Jr: Comparison of cerebrovascular response to hypoxic and carbon monoxide hypoxia in newborn and adult sheep. J Cerebral Blood Flow and Metab 4:115–122, 1984
8. Jones MD, Rosenberg AA, Koehler RC, Traystman RJ, Simmons MA, Molteni RA: Oxygen delivery to the brain before and after birth. Science 216:324–325, 1982
9. Koehler RC, Jones MD, Traystman RJ: Cerebral circulatory response to carbon monoxide and hypoxic hypoxia in the lamb. Am J Physiol 243:H27–H32, 1982
10. Jones MD Jr, Rosenberg AA, Traystman RJ, Koehler RC: Oxyhemoglobin dissociation and cerebral O_2 delivery in fetal sheep. Fed Proc 41:1527, 1982
11. Berne RM, Winn HR, Rubio R: The local regulation of cerebral blood flow. Prog Cardiovasc Dis 24:243–260, 1981
12. Kontos HA, Wei EP, Raper AJ, Rosenblum WI, Navari RM, Patterson JL Jr: Role of tissue hypoxia in local regulation of cerebral microcirculation. Am J Physiol 234:H582–H591, 1978
13. Koehler RC, Traystman RJ, Rosenberg AA, Hudak ML, Jones MD Jr: Role of O_2-hemoglobin affinity in cerebrovascular response to carbon monoxide hypoxia. Am J Physiol H1019–H1023, 1983
14. Battaglia FC, McGaughey H, Makowski EL, Meschia G: Postnatal changes in oxygen affinity of sheep red cells: a dual role of diphosphoglyceric acid. Am J Physiol 219:217–221, 1970
15. Bard H, Teasdale F: Red cell oxygen affinity, hemoglobin type, 2,3-diphosphoglycerate, and pH as a function of fetal development. Pediatrics 64:483–487, 1979
16. Wade JPH, du Boulay GH, Marshall J, Pearson TC, Ross Russell RW, Shirley JA, Symon L, Wetherly-Mein G, Zilkha E. Cerebral blood flow, haematocrit and viscosity in subjects with a high oxygen affinity haemoglobin variant. Acta Neurol Scand 61:210–215, 1980

17. Jones MD Jr, Sheldon RE, Peeters LL, Makowski EL, Meschia G: Regulation of cerebral blood flow in the ovine fetus. Am J Physiol 235:162–166, 1978

18. Ashwal S, Majcher JS, Longo LD: Patterns of fetal lamb regional cerebral blood flow during and after prolonged hypoxia: studies during the posthypoxic recovery period. Am J Obstet Gynecol 139:365–372, 1981

19. Borgstrom LH, Johannsson H, Siesjo BK: The influence of acute normovolemic anemia on cerebral blood flow and oxygen consumption of anesthetized rats. Acta Physiol Scand 93:505–514, 1975

20. Fumia FD, Edelstone DI, Caritis SN, Mueller-Heubach EM: Relationship of O_2 delivery and blood flow to arterial O_2 content (CaO_2) in fetal lambs: effects of isovolemic anemia and polycythemia. In: Proceedings of the 29th Annual Meeting of the Society for Gynecologic Investigation. p 125, 1982

21. Paulson OB, Parving HH, Olesen J, and Skinhoj E: Influence of carbon monoxide and of hemodilution on cerebral blood flow and blood gases in man. J Appl Physiol 35:111–116, 1973

22. Doblar DD, Santiago TV, Edelman NH: Correlation between ventilatory and cerebrovascular responses to inhalation of CO J Appl Physiol 43:455–462, 1977

23. Roughton FJW: Transport of organ and carbon dioxide. In: Handbook of Physiology. Respiration. Vol 1. American Physiological Society, Washington, pp 767–825, 1964

24. Traystman RJ, Fitzgerald RS, Loscutoff SC: Cerebral circulatory responses to arterial hypoxia in normal and chemodenervated dogs. Circ Res 42:649–657, 1978

25. Mahler HR, Cordes EH: Biological oxidations. In: Biological Chemistry, 2nd Ed, Harper & Row Publishers, New York, p 631–711, 1966

26. Wright GR, Shepard RJ: Physiological effect of carbon monoxide. In: Robertshaw D (ed), International Review of Physiology. Environmental Physiology III, Vol 20. University Park Press, Baltimore, pp 311–368, 1979

27. Savolainen H, Kurppa K, Tenhunen R, Kivisto H: Biochemical effects of carbon monoxide poisoning in rat brain with special reference to blood carboxyhemoglobin and cerebral cytochrome oxidase activity. Neurosci Lett 19:319–323, 1980

28. Fujishima M, Scheinberg P, Busto R, Reinmuth OM: The relation between cerebral oxygen consumption and cerebral vascular reactivity to carbon dioxide. Stroke 2:251–257, 1971

29. Hernandez MJ, Brennan RW, Vannucci RC, Bowman GS: Cerebral blood flow and oxygen consumption in the newborn dog. Am J Physiol 234:R209–R215, 1978

30. Reivich M, Brann AW Jr, Shapiro H, Rawson J, Sano N: Reactivity of cerebral vessels to CO_2 in the newborn rhesus monkey. Eur Neurol 6:132–136, 1971/1972

31. Rosenberg AA, Jones MD Jr, Traystman RJ, Simmons MA, Molteni RA: Response of cerebral flood flow to changes in PCO_2 in fetal, newborn, and adult sheep. Am J Physiol 242:H862–H866, 1982

32. Kontos HA, Raper AJ, Patterson JL Jr: Analysis of vasoactivity of local pH, PCO_2 and bicarbonate on pial vessels. Stroke 8:358–360, 1977

33. Kety SS, Schmidt CF: The determination of cerebral blood flow in man by the use of nitrous oxide in low concentrations. Am J Physiol 143:53–56, 1945

34. Purves MJ: The Physiology of the Cerebral Circulation. Cambridge University Press, London, 1972

35. Todd MM, Shapiro HM, Obrist WD: Cerebral blood flow measurements in the critically ill patient. In: Grenvik A, Safar P (ed), Brain Failure and Resuscitation. Churchill Livingstone, New York, pp 125–154, 1981

36. Cold GE, Jensen FT: Cerebral blood flow in the acute phase after head injury. Part 1: Correlation to age of the patients, clinical outcome and localization of the infused region. Acta Anaesth Scand 24:245–251, 1980

37. Donegan JM, Koehler RC, Jones MD Jr, Rogers MC, Traystman RJ: Effect of reduced cerebral O_2 consumption on the cerebrovascular response to hypoxia. Physiologist 24:77, 1981

38. Smith AL: Effect of anesthetics and oxygen deprivation on brain blood flow and metabolism. Surg Clin North Am 55:819–837, 1975
39. Smith, FW: Nuclear magnetic resonance in the investigation of cerebral disorder. J Cerebral Blood Flow and Metab 3:263–269, 1983
40. Greenberg RP, Ward JD, Lutz H, Miller JD, Becker DP: Advanced monitoring of the brain. In: Grenvik A, Safar P (ed), Brain Failure and Resuscitation. Churchill Livingstone, New York, pp 67–90, 1981

4. SURFACTANT TURNOVER, SURFACTANT THERAPY, AND THE DEVELOPING LUNG

Alan Jobe

INTRODUCTION

I will summarize the new concepts concerning the metabolism of surfactant, the available information on the physiologic and biochemical effects of surfactant therapy, and some unique features of the developing lung that influence the strategies used to treat lung disease in the infant. While these observations are directed toward the responses of the immature lung to ventilation, the same events no doubt occur in the mature lung in disease, although their relative importance has not been defined. A developmental perspective toward lung disease and its therapy is a rewarding approach that will yield insight into the processes of lung disease in the older child and adult.

SURFACTANT METABOLISM, AN OVERVIEW

Surfactant is a complex array of primarily phospholipids and a specific apoprotein that together have unique surface tension lowering properties (1). While the composition of surfactant is important for biophysical function, the structure of the three-dimensional surface macroaggregate is critical. The surfactant complex is synthesized only by type II epithelial cells which occupy only about 7% of the surface area of the alveolus and are about 16% of the lung cells in the adult human lung (2). Synthesis of the various components of the surfactant complex occurs in the endoplasmic reticulum, and, in general, the synthetic pathways are those common to all mammalian cells (1). The unique process related to surfactant metabolism is the translocation and condensation of the surfactant components into the secretory organelles, the lammellar bodies (3, 4). The mechanisms by which the type II cell can generate these dense, highly ordered, lipid aggregates remain to be defined. However, the kinetics of the movement of phospholipid components from the endoplasmic reticulum to lamellar bodies, and subsequently to the alveoli can be measured following the injection of radiolabeled precursors in vivo. Early studies reported only the decay kinetics of the labeling of saturated or total phosphatidylcholine from lung tissue or the alveoli (5–8).

The biological half-life of surfactant phosphatidylcholine was found to be 15–20 hr. However, these estimates do not accurately reflect the very dynamic metabolic characteristics of surfactant phosphatidylcholine, because assumptions of a biological half-life measurement were not satisfied by the metabolism of surfactant (9). Alveolar surfactant is not pulse labeled following the intravascular injection of labeled phospholipid precursors (Figure 1). The time to reach a maximal specific activity in alveolar phosphatidylcholine is 6 to 8 hr in adult rabbits and almost 20 hr in 3-day old rabbits (10). Thus, alveolar surfactant cannot be pulse labeled by intravascular injections of labeled precursors. Using a two component model for surfactant metabolism that is independent of pulse labeling or reutilization (see below), the lamellar bodies can be shown to be the precursors of alveolar surfactant, and a turnover time can be calculated (10). The turnover is the time necessary to refill the alveolar surfactant pool of it were empty. The turnover time of alveolar phosphatidylcholine in adult rabbits and rats was estimated to be 3–10 hr by different laboratories (10, 11, 12). Three-day old rabbits were found to have turnover times about 3 times longer than adult rabbits (10 hr vs 3 hr), but these young rabbits had larger surfactant pool sizes and therefore larger hourly flux rates of surfactant phosphatidylcholine from lamellar bodies to the alveoli (10).

A second problem with the biological half-life measurement is that surfactant is reutilized. Based on the conservation of labeled phospholipids with time and the close correspondence of specific activities of phosphatidylcholine in the lamellar

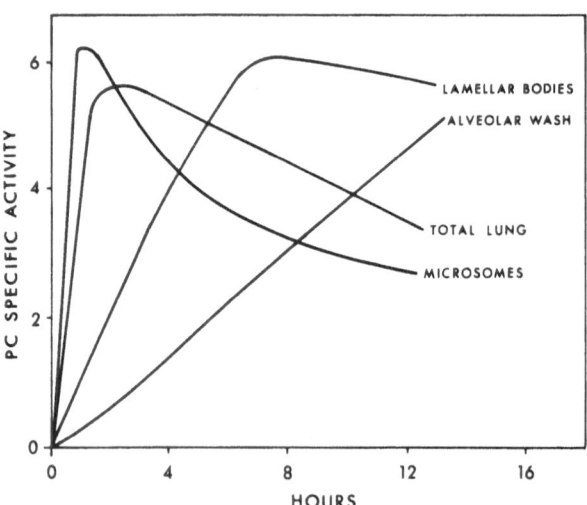

Figure 1. Specific activity–time relationships of phosphatidylcholine. Specific activities of phosphatidylcholine (PC) in subcellular fractions from adult rabbit lung were measured following an intravascular injection of radiolabeled choline. The radiolabeled phosphatidylcholine sequentially is recovered from microsomal, lamellar body and alveolar wash fractions. The curves have been sketched from Ref. 8–10.

bodies and alveoli at late times, one can deduce that the labeled phosphatidylcholine is recycled back into lamellar bodies for resecretion (9, 10). This process will be referred to as reutilization. Reutilization has been demonstrated directly by the measurement of uptake by lamellar bodies of radiolabeled natural surfactant following intratracheal injection (13, 14). Using this approach, we have measured an efficiency of reutilization of surfactant phosphatidylcholine in 3-day old rabbits of about 95% (14). De novo synthesis contributes only about 5% to the hourly flux of surfactant between the lamellar bodies and the alveoli, and at equilibrium catabolism just balances de novo synthesis, and therefore is a relatively minor component in the metabolic equation. Thus, the dominant pathway in surfactant metabolism is the reutilization pathway. While magnitude of reutilization has not been measured to date in adult animals, the process certainly occurs (13–15).

The mechanism by which surfactant is reprocessed by the type II cell likely is a process of bulk uptake not unlike endocytosis. Williams has demonstrated uptake of both cationic ferritin and a lectin that specifically binds to the apical plasma membrane of type II cells (16, 17). These proteins were found initially in multivesicular bodies and subsequently they became associated with the non lamellar protein containing areas of the lamellar bodies. Phosphatidylcholine is reutilized intact and without degradative and synthetic steps (13, 14). Jacobs et al. (18) has documented no structural specificity for phosphatidylcholine by using specific analogues of phosphatidylcholine. However, the efficiency of reutilization and clearance from the lung clearly differs depending on what form of surfactant or lipid complex is administered by tracheal injection and possibly on species and age of the animals that are studied (Table 1).

We must view surfactant metabolism as a very dynamic metabolic process that includes a reutilization pathway that likely dominates the flux of surfactant between the type II cell and the alveolus. The metabolic characteristics of the system must be important for function. Surfactant can be readily inactivated in vivo by hyperventilation or by aggregation with atelectasis (24–26). Surfactant pool sizes also increase acutely with exercise (27). Magoon et al. have fractionated the alveolar surfactant into a series of pools that they feel represent the sequence from secretion to reutilization (15). We assume that since the major component of surfactant, phosphatidylcholine, is reutilized intact, the process of reutilization probably is important for the maintenance of the 3-dimensional structure of the macroaggregate for optimal surface tension lowering behavior. Thus, reutilization 'reactivates' surfactant without requiring the very energy expensive de novo synthesis of new lipids. This dynamic, cyclic process may be disrupted in presently unsuspected ways in disease.

Table 1. Recovery of labeled phospholipid following tracheal injection.

Phospholipid aggregate	Animal	Dose as % of surfactant pool size	% of dose remaining at 6 hours		Reference
			Alveolar wash	Alveolar wash + lung	
PC[a] complexed to albumin	Fetal lamb	>1%	10% (at 1.5 hr)	—	Scarpelli et al. (19)
Nebulized DPPC[b]	Rat	>1%	—	25%	Geiger et al. (20)
Lyophilized and homogenized surfactant	Adult rabbit	4%	8%	50%	Hallman et al. (13)
Liposomes of DPPC	Adult rabbit	5–7%	40%	60%	Oyarzun et al. (21)
Liposomes of DPPC + PG[c]	Adult rabbit	5–7%	25%	60%	Oyarzun et al. (21)
Natural surfactant	3-day old rabbit	5–10%	40%	75%	Jacobs et al. (14)
Natural surfactant	newborn lamb	20%	45%	85%	Glatz et al. (22)
Natural surfactant	3-day old rabbit	450%	40%	80%	Oguchi et al. (23)
Liposomes of DPPC	3-day old rabbit	400%	70%	85%	Oguchi et al. (23)

[a] PC is phosphatidylcholine.
[b] DPPC is dipalmitoylphosphatidylcholine.
[c] PG is phosphatidylglycerol.

Surfactant metabolism and surfactant replacement in the developing lung

The developing lung of the human stores increasing amounts of surfactant within lung tissue from about 20 weeks gestational age (28). Synthetic pathways must be present at that early date. Some infants born at 25 to 26 weeks gestational age do not have lung disease characterized by surfactant deficiency, demonstrating that the human lung has an approx. 10-week window during which 'early' maturation can occur. My view is that this early maturation represents the development of secretory potential rather than synthetic potential. During labor and following term or premature birth, an animal releases the tissue stores of surfactant to the alveoli (29). We have documented that prematurely delivered lambs secrete their surfactant stores within several hours of birth, and the kinetics of secretion is independent of the final pool size achieved (30). Following this initial release of surfactant, the surfactant pool size does not increase very much. This initial secretory burst must be quantitatively sufficient to permit pulmonary adaptation if respiratory distress syndrome (RDS) is to be prevented. De novo synthesis cannot acutely augment the surfactant pool size for two reasons. 1. The hourly rate of synthesis is small relative to the overall flux of surfactant (14). 2. The time delays from synthesis to secretion are very long in developing animals (10). Following the intravascular injection of radiolabeled palmitic acid in newborn lambs, the specific activity of alveolar surfactant-associated dipalmitoylphosphatidylcholine from the de novo synthetic pathway was not maximal for at least 24 hr (31) (Figure 2). Similarly measured maximal specific activities in ventilated premature lambs with an RDS-like syndrome were not achieved until at least 30 hr after precursor injection (32). However, once surfactant is present within the alveolus of the healthy newborn, it remains there for a very long time. Following the administration of radiolabeled surfactant to term lambs at birth, about 40% of the surfactant became lung tissue associated and the rest remained within the alveoli. The pattern of association was consistent with reutilization and the labeled surfactant was cleared from the lung compartment (alveolar wash + lung tissue) with a biological half-life of 6 days (22).

The alveolar pool size of surfactant/kg is about 3 times larger following neonatal adaption in the term newborn than in the adult (33). This large pool size decreases linearly over 12 days in the rabbit to become equivalent on a body weight basis to that measured in the adult (33). The physiologic reason for a large surfactant pool size is not known. The pool size of surfactant in prematurely delivered and ventilated lambs with severe RDS was about 15% to 75% that measured in healthy term lambs, and the severity of RDS correlated with surfactant pool size (34). Thus, some premature lambs with RDS have a surfactant pool size that is quantitatively similar to the adult when expressed as pool size/kg body weight. However, the intratracheal administration of 50 mg natural surfactant

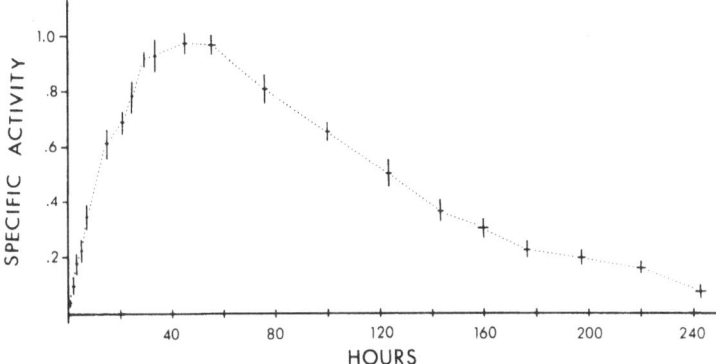

Figure 2. Labeling of saturated phosphatidylcholine recovered from airways of term newborn lambs. The specific activities (cpm/μmol phosphate) of saturated phosphatidylcholine in samples recovered by an airway suction technique from the airways of 7 newborn lambs following the intravascular injection of [³H] palmitic acid are expressed as a fraction of the maximal specific activities achieved versus time after isotope injection. Figure reproduced from Ref. 31 with permission.

lipid/kg will improve lung function in these lambs, demonstrating a functional surfactant deficiency (32, 35).

The effect of the intratracheal administration of 60 to 140 mg surfactant lipid/kg (doses comparable to those used in clinical trials) on endogenous surfactant metabolism in the developing lung has not been carefully studied. Stewart-De Haan reported no effect of surfactant administration on the incorporation of radiolabeled glycerol and palmitic acid into the lung lipids of newborn rabbits (36). We have documented saturated phosphatidylcholine synthesis and secretion following delivery, treatment with surfactant, and ventilation of premature lambs over a period of several days (32). Similarly, the intratracheal injection into 3-day old rabbits of amounts of natural surfactant that were about 4.5 times the endogenous pool size did not decrease the incorporation of labeled palmitic acid, choline or ^{32}P into lung phosphatidylcholine (23). The amount of labeled phosphatidylcholine that was secreted also was not changed, and the rabbits continued to increase their alveolar pool size despite the presence of large amounts of exogenously administered surfactant within their lungs (23). No adverse biochemical effects of the exogenous administration of surfactant have been documented in the few animal studies that have been reported.

The acute and chronic effects of surfactant on cardiopulmonary function in the premature infant also have not been well studied. Following the tracheal administration of natural sheep surfactant suspended in 15 ml fluid to prematurely delivered and ventilated lambs at 135 days gestational age, cardiac outputs, systemic artery pressures, pulmonary artery pressures, and ductal shunts did not change when compared to pretreatment values (35). Thus, no apparent cardiovascular compromise resulted from the instillation of a relatively large volume of suspension into the airways of these premature lambs. However, in more immature lambs delivered and ventilated at 120 days gestational age, surfactant treatment caused a drop in pulmonary vascular resistance with a resulting increase in the left to right ductal shunt (37). These different results probably reflect different responses of the pulmonary vasculature at different maturational stages.

The distribution of surfactant to the lungs also will affect response. If surfactant is mixed with fetal lung fluid at birth, a rather uniform distribution of the surfactant throughout the lung can be achieved (38). However, instillation after the onset of ventilation resulted in a very nonhomogeneous distribution pattern. Following treatment and 20 min of ventilation, the aerated volumes of such lungs were found to contain 5·4 times more surfactant than the atelectatic volumes. Surprisingly, following surfactant instillation, pulmonary blood flow distribution changed from being very uniform throughout the lungs to a pattern of distribution characterized by a relative fall in blood flow to aerated lung volumes and an increase to atelectatic volumes of lungs in these premature lambs. We postulate that the nonhomogeneous distribution of surfactant will result in a wide range of compliance changes throughout the lung. In fully aerated areas the peak inspiratory pressures of 28–31 cm H_2O may be transmitted to the pulmonary micro-vasculature and inhibit blood flow. In fact, significant overdistension and air trapping may occur in areas receiving large amounts of surfactant. In areas of low compliance, there may be very little pressure transmitted from the airways to the pulmonary microvasculature. These observations of ductal flows and pulmonary perfusion suggest that unexpected cardiopulmonary responses may occur following surfactant instillation and acute changes in arterial blood gas values.

Surfactant quantity versus surfactant function

A consistent observation following the treatment of very premature lambs and some infants with surfactant is that the response decreases with time after treatment (39–41). The duration of response is longer for lambs treated at birth than for lambs treated after a period of ventilation (42). Since much of the surfactant appears to remain within the airways for a long time, an explanation other than clearance of the surfactant is needed. As developed above, the aggregate structure of surfactant is critical for surface function and the preservation of function may depend on ventilatory patterns and recycling processes. These possibilities have not been evaluated in the lung with RDS. However, the immature structure of the lung of the premature contributes indirectly to surfactant dysfunction in the premature. Nilsson et al. (43) describe the rapid development of bronchiolar epithelial disruption following ventilation of premature rabbit lungs. Surfactant therapy before the onset of ventilation prevents the development of this lesion (43). Hyaline membranes result from the coagulation of intra-alveolar proteins and cellular debris. Thus, the epithelial integrity of the immature lung can be disrupted by ventilation and proteinaceous fluid can enter the airways. Coagulation in vitro will trap about 50% of the surfactant that is in suspension (44), and soluble proteins can interfere with the surface tension lowering properties of surfactant (45, 46). The amount of protein recovered by alveolar wash from the alveoli of prematurely delivered and ventilated lambs increased by 60 mg/kg hr (Figure 3) (47). That increase in protein resulted from a bidirectional flux of protein from the alveoli to the vascular space and from the vascular space to the alveoli. The amount of the protein leak was linearly correlated with the peak inspiratory pressures (or mean airway pressures) needed to normalize the blood gas values of the lambs (47). Thus, the protein leak increased as the severity of the lung disease increased. Three factors have been identified which affect the magnitude of the protein leak. 1. If premature lambs (120 or 135 days gestational age) and term lambs are ventilated with equivalent pressures and equivalent blood gases are achieved, the protein leak is about four-fold higher in the premature lung (48). 2. If premature lambs are treated with surfactant, the protein leak can be significantly decreased (Figure 3). 3. The ventilation of the premature lung results in epithelial disruption and the magni-

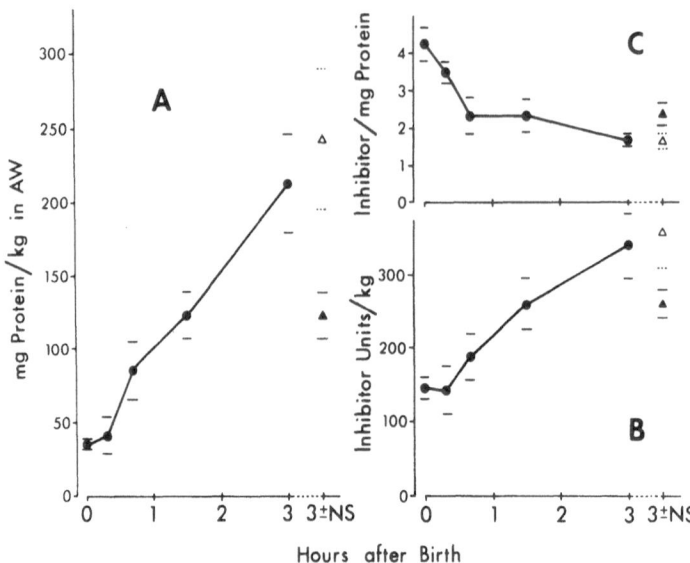

Figure 3. Amount of protein and inhibitor of surfactant recovered in alveolar washes from prematurely delivered and ventilated lambs. A: Mean ± SE values of mg protein/kg recovered by alveolar wash from lambs sacrificed at times from delivery to 3 hr of age (●——●). Slope of the least-squares regression line fit to the data was 60 mg/kg hr (R = 0.893). Values for 8 twin pairs of lambs that were treated (+NS, ▲) or not treated with surfactant at birth (–NS, △) and ventilated for 3 hr are also shown. B: Amount of inhibitory activity of the surface tension lowering characteristics of sheep surfactant in the soluble protein phase of alveolar washes was titrated. C: Ratio of inhibitor unit/kg to mg protein/kg was calculated for the 3 groups of lambs. Symbols are as in frames A and B. Figure reproduced from Ref. 47 with permission.

tude of the protein leak increases as ventilatory pressures increase.

The protein leak and the epithelial disruption will result in hyaline membrane formation and at least some sequestration of surfactant within the hyaline membranes. Albumin and globulins do not interfere with the surface tension lowering properties of surfactant, but alveolar washes from prematurely delivered and ventilated lambs contain a protein that at very low concentrations disrupts surfactant function in vitro (Figure 3) (49). This protein has been purified from the alveolar washes from lambs; it is an approx. 110 000 MW dimer that interacts reversibly at low concentrations with surfactant to raise minimum surface tension, increase the time of spreading and adsorption of surfactant to a surface, and increase the area of surface compression needed to lower surface tensions (50). A similar protein has been isolated from the airways of premature infants with RDS, and its presence has been correlated with high surface tensions in surfactant samples from these infants (51).

CONCLUSIONS

The metabolism of surfactant is very complex and dynamic, and the intricacies of that metabolism remain to be delineated in both the adult and immature lung. However, the process of reutilization likely is critical for the maintenance of an adequate surfactant pool size, and acute changes in surfactant pools no doubt result primarily from shifts in the recycling pathways. De novo synthesis and degradation probably contribute only to the relatively long-term regulation of surfactant pools. Surfactant function in the immature lung or by extrapolation in the diseased lung of the older child and adult depends upon not only the adequacy of the alveolar pool size of surfactant but also the functional adequacy of the surfactant. Thus, surfactant dysfunction can result from inadequate pool sizes, ineffective reprocessing, sequestration within hyaline membranes, or functional inhibition by soluble proteins within the alveolus. The quantitative contributions of these and possibly other factors in different diseases remain to be defined.

ACKNOWLEDGEMENT

This work was supported by grants HD-12714 and HD-11932 from the Departments of Health and Human Development.

REFERENCES

1. Van Golde LMG: Metabolism of phospholipids in the lung. Am Rev Respir Dis 114:977–1000, 1976
2. Crapo JD, Barry BE, Gehr P, Bachofen M, Weibel ER: Number and cell characteristics of the normal human lung. Am Rev Respir Dis 125:322–337, 1982
3. Jobe A, Ikegami M, Sarton-Miller I, Jones S, Yu G: Characterization of phospholipids and localization of some phospholipid synthetic and subcellular marker enzymes in subcellular fractions from rabbit lung. Biochim Biophys Acta 666:47–57, 1981
4. Okazaki T, Johnston JM, Snyder JM: Morphogenesis of the lamellar body in fetal lung tissue in vitro. Biochim Biophys Acta 712:283–291, 1982
5. Tierney DF, Clements JA, Trahan HJ: Rates of replacement of lecithins and alveolar instability in rat lungs. Am J Physiol 213:671–676, 1967
6. Young SL, Tierney DF: Dipalmitoyl lecithin secretion and metabolism by the rat lung. Am J Physiol 222:1539–1544, 1972
7. Toshima N, Akino T, Ohno K: Turnover time of lecithin in lung tissue and alveolar wash of rat. Tohoku J Exp Med 108:265–277, 1972
8. Jobe A: The labeling and biological half-life of phosphatidylcholine in subcellular fractions of rabbit lung. Biochim Biophys Acta 489:440–453, 1977
9. Jobe AH, Jacobs HC: Catabolism of pulmonary surfactant. In: Robertson, Batenburg, Van Golde (eds), Pulmonary Surfactant. Elsevier/North Holland Medical Press (in press)
10. Jacobs H, Jobe A, Ikegami M, Jones S: Surfactant phosphatidylcholine source, fluxes, and turnover times in 3-day old, 10-day old and adult rabbits. J Biol Chem 257:1805–1810, 1982

60

11. Baritussio AG, Magoon MW, Goerke J, Clements JA: Precursor-product relationship between rabbit type II cell lamellar bodies and alveolar surface-active material. Biochim Biophys Acta 666:382–393, 1981

12. Young SL, Kremers SA, Apple JS, Crapo JD, Brumley GW: Rat lung surfactant kinetics: biochemical and morphometric correlation. J Appl Physiol 51:248–253, 1981

13. Hillman M, Epstein BL, Gluck L: Analysis of labeling and clearance of lung surfactant phospholipids in rabbit. Evidence of bidirectional surfactant flux between lamellar bodies and alveolar lavage. J Clin Invest 68:742–751, 1981

14. Jacobs H, Jobe A, Ikegami M, Conaway D: The significance of reutilization of surfactant phosphatidylcholine. J Biol Chem 258:4159–4165, 1983

15. Magoon MW, Wright JR, Baritussio A, Williams MC, Goerke J, Benson BJ, Hamilton RL, Clements JA: Subfractionation of lung surfactant. Biochim Biophys Acta 750:18–31, 1983

16. Williams MC: A possible endocytic pathway for return of secreted surfactant to lamellar bodies. J Cell Biol 95:388A, 1982

17. Williams MC: Uptake of MPA-ferritin by alveolar type II cells in vivo. Am Rev Respir Dis 127:271, 1983

18. Jacobs H, Jobe A, Ikegami M: Specificity of reutilization of surfactant phosphatidylcholine in rabbits. Am Rev Respir Dis 127:276, 1983

19. Scarpelli EM, Condorelli S, Colacicco G, Cosmi EV: Lamb fetal pulmonary fluid. II. Fate of phosphatidylcholine. Pediatr Res 9:195–201, 1975

20. Geiger K, Gallagher ML, Hedley-Whyte J: Cellular distribution and clearance of aerosolized dipalmitoyl lecithin. J Appl Physiol 39:759–766, 1975

21. Oyarzun MJ, Clements JA, Baritussio A: Ventilation enhances pulmonary alveolar clearance of radioactive dipalmitoyl phosphatidylcholine in liposomes. Am Rev Respir Dis 121:709–721, 1980

22. Glatz T, Ikegami M, Jobe A: Metabolism of exogenously administered natural surfactant in the newborn lamb. Pediatr Res 16:711–715, 1982

23. Oguchi K, Ikegami M, Jacobs HC, Jobe AH: Clearance of large amounts of natural surfactant and dipalmitoylphosphatidylcholine from the lungs of 3-day old rabbits following tracheal injection. Clin Res 32:126A, 1984

24. Wyszogrodski I, Kyei-Aboagye K, Taeusch HW Jr, Avery ME: Surfactant inactivation by hyperventilation: conservation by end-expiratory pressure. J Appl Physiol 38:461–466, 1975

25. Thet LA, Clerch L, Massaro GD, Massaro D: Changes in sedimentation of surfactant in ventilated excised rat lungs. J Clin Invest 64:600–608, 1979

26. Massaro D, Clerch L, Temple D, Baier H: Surfactant deficiency in rats without a decreased amount of extracellular surfactant. J Clin Invest 71:1536–1543, 1983

27. Nicholas TE, Power JHT, Barr HA: Surfactant homeostasis in the rat lung during swimming exercise. J Appl Physiol 53:1521–1528, 1982

28. Clements JA, Tooley WH: Kinetics of surface-active material in the fetal lung. In: Hodson WA (ed), Development of the Lung. Marcel Dekker, New York, pp 349–366, 1977

29. Rooney SA, Gobran LI, Wai-Lee TS: Stimulation of surfactant production by oxytocin-induced labor in the rabbit. J Clin Invest 60:754, 1977

30. Jacobs H, Jobe A, Ikegami M, Jones S: How lambs with RDS accumulate a surfactant pool with time. Pediatr Res 16:292A, 1982

31. Ikegami M, Jobe A, Nathanielsz PW: The labeling of pulmonary surfactant phosphatidylcholine in newborn and adult sheep. Exp Lung Res 2:197–206, 1981

32. Jobe A, Ikegami M, Glatz T, Yoshida Y, Diakomanolis E, Padbury J: Saturated phosphatidylcholine secretion and the effect of natural surfactant on premature and term lambs ventilated for 2 days. Exp Lung Res 4:259–267, 1983

33. Jobe A, Ikegami M, Jacobs H: Changes in the amount of lung and airway phosphatidylcholine in 0.5–12.5-day old rabbits. Biochim Biophys Acta 664:182–187, 1981

34. Jobe AH, Ikegami M, Jacobs HC, Jones SJ: Surfactant pool sizes and severity of respiratory

distress syndrome in prematurely delivered lambs. Am Rev Respir Dis 127:751–755, 1983

35. Jobe A, Jacobs H, Ikegami M, Jones S: Cardiovascular effects of surfactant suspensions given by tracheal instillation to premature lambs. Pediatr Res 17:444–448, 1983

36. Stewart-De Haan PJ, Metcalfe IL, Harding PGR, Enhorning G, Possmayer F: Effect of birth and surfactant treatment on phospholipid synthesis in the premature rabbit. Biol Neonate 38:238–247, 1980

37. Clyman RI, Jobe A, Heymann M, Ikegami M, Roman C, Payne B, Mauray F: Increased shunt through the patent ductus arteriosus after surfactant replacement therapy. J Pediatr 100:101–107, 1982

38. Jobe A, Jacobs H, Ikegami M, Jones S: Distribution of surfactant and pulmonary blood flow following surfactant treatment of premature lambs. Pediatr Res 17:319A, 1983

39. Jacobs H, Jobe A, Ikegami M, Glatz T, Jones, SJ, Barajas L: Premature lambs rescued from respiratory failure with natural surfactant: clinical and biophysical correlates. Pediatr Res 16:424–429, 1982

40. Hallman M, Merritt TA, Schneider H, Epstein BL, Mannino F, Edwards DK, Gluck L: Isolation of human surfactant from amniotic fluid and a pilot study of its efficacy in respiratory distress syndrome. Pediatrics 71:473–482, 1983

41. Smyth JA, Metcalfe IL, Duffty P, Possmayer F, Bryan MH, Enhorning G: Hyaline membrane disease treated with bovine surfactant. Pediatrics 71:913–917, 1983

42. Jobe A, Ikegami M, Glatz T, Yoshida Y, Diakomanolis E, Padbury J: Duration and characteristcs of treatment of premature lambs with natural surfactant. J Clin Invest 67:370–375, 1981

43. Nilsson R, Grossman G, Robertson B: Lung surfactant and the pathogenesis of neonatal broncheolar lesions induced by artificial ventilation. Pediatr Res 12:249–255, 1978

44. Balis J, Shelley S, McCue M, Rappaport E: Mehanisms of damage to the lung surfactant system. Exp Mol Pathol 14:243–262, 1971

45. Taylor FB, Abrams ME: Effect of surface active lipoprotein on clotting and fibrinolysis, and of fibrinogen on surface tension of surface active lipoprotein. Am J Med 40:346–350, 1966

46. Tierney DF, Johnson RP: Altered surface tension of lung extracts and lung mechanics. J Appl Physiol 20:1253–1260, 1965

47. Jobe A, Ikegami M, Jacobs H, Jones S, Conaway D: Permeability of premature lamb lungs to protein and the effect of surfactant on that permeability. J Appl Physiol 55:169–176, 1983

48. Jobe A, Ikegami M, Jacobs H: Increased lung protein permeability of prematurely delivered and ventilated lambs. Clin Res 32:132A, 1984

49. Ikegami M, Jobe A, Glatz T: Surface activity following natural surfactant treatment in premature lambs. J Appl Physiol 51:306–312, 1981

50. Ikegami M, Jobe A, Jacobs H: Some properties of a purified inhibitor of surfactant function. Am Rev Respir Dis 127:212, 1983

51. Ikegami M, Jacobs H, Jobe A: Surfactant function in respiratory distress syndrome. J Pediatr 102:443–447, 1983

5. SURFACTANT SUPPLEMENTATION

GORAN ENHORNING

Not until late in gestation does surfactant (SA) synthesis become adequate, allowing a smooth transition from intra- to extrauterine life. If delivery is too early, there would be an SA deficiency, which quite likely would result in the development of the respiratory distress syndrome (RDS). The first breath would then meet excessive resistance, but if the lungs became expanded in spite of this, air distribution would be uneven and the airways would tend to close again during expiration. The neonate obviously would never encounter these difficulties if the SA deficiency were compensated for by an instillation of pulmonary SA before the first attempt to aerate the lungs. This concept of supplementing the SA the instant before it is needed was not put to the test until 1972. Enhorning and Robertson (1) reported that lung compliance in rabbits delivered on the 27th day of gestation, when SA synthesis is still very inadequate, improved dramatically following instillation of SA into the trachea. This was the first in a series of animal experiments (2–6) demonstrating the efficacy of SA supplementation prior to the first breath.

The key to our success was the use of natural SA. We had found that no other product than the SA originating from mature lungs had the physical properties we believed were necessary for successful supplementation. We evaluated the various products considered for this purpose with the pulsating bubble technique (7, 8), which simulates the events of the first breath. A small sample chamber filled with the liquid to be tested communicates with ambient air through a narrow capillary. As some of the liquid is withdrawn, the first breath is simulated. Air moves down the airway until a bubble expands at the lower tip of the capillary. The bubble, the 'alveolus', is maintained at a specific size ($r = 0.55$ mm) for 10 sec, following which a pulsator initiates 'breathing' by moving liquid in and out of the chamber. The bubble then oscillates at a rate of 20 rpm from a maximal to a minimal size ($r = 0.55$ mm and 0.4 mm, respectively). Throughout this procedure which, including 10 cycles, takes less than one minute, the pressure around the bubble is measured. The pressure difference, ΔP, at the air–liquid interface is obtained and, since the bubble radius, r, is known, it is possible to calculate surface tension, γ, from the law of Laplace, $\Delta P = 2\gamma/r$.

Using this mode of assessment, it was found that the SA in the airway fluid of a fetus at term, or in the lungs of an adult animal, has certain characteristics which probably are essential for successful lung expansion. Adsorption of amphipathic phospholipid molecules to the air–liquid interface is extremely fast, since the pressure tracing indicates that, as soon as the bubble has been expanded, a monomolecular layer forms in the bubble surface, lowering surface tension from the value characterizing water at 37° C, 70 mN/m, to approximately 25 mN/m. When pulsation has begun, surface tension of close to zero is reached the first time the bubble is compressed to minimal size. A direct inspection of the pressure tracing shows that the transmural pressure necessary to overcome the effect of surface tension is being reduced as the bubble decreases in size during 'expiration'. This truly illustrates the stabilizing effect of SA.

The pulsating bubble surfactometer requires such a small volume of fluid that the liquid in the airways of fetal rabbits can be studied. At a gestational age of 26 days, the rabbit clearly has an SA deficiency. At 27 days, there is more SA available in the airways and, if delivered on that day, some rabbit pups are able to expand their lungs and survive for a few hours. One day later, the airway fluid has much better surface properties, and chances for survival if delivered on the 29th day are quite good. However, it is not until the 30th day that SA is present in abundance in the airway fluid and, on that day, aeration is seemingly very simple, requiring minimal effort.

A lung lavage from adult animals yields a suspension with surface properties very similar to those of the airway fluid of a fetus at term. By simple centrifugation procedures, the SA of the lavage fluid can be concentrated. It was the crude SA, obtained from lung lavage of young adult rabbits, at a phospholipid concentration of 10–20 mg/ml, that was used in most of our early animal studies. Clearly, this was a preparation unacceptable for use in human neonates.

The first attempts to supplement the newborn infant's inadequate SA stores were not particularly successful (9, 10). We can now understand why. Only dipalmitoylphosphatidylcholine (DPPC), the main component of SA, was administered and, alone, this phospholipid adsorbs extremely slowly to the air–liquid interface. The liposomes the DPPC forms when suspended in water are probably very stable, so much so that they will not break up to form a monolayer at the air–liquid interface. DPPC is possibly the only component of the compressed final monolayer at the air–liquid interface (11) but, for this phospholipid to form a monomolecular layer, other phospholipids and possibly proteins are needed. Natural SA has the ability to adsorb quickly, and this property is not lost when the lipids are extracted with chloroform-methanol and then resuspended in saline. Fujiwara (12) was the first to use such an extract of natural SA to treat human infants. His preparation was of bovine origin and was reinforced with synthetic DPPC and phosphatidylglycerol (PG) in a molar ratio of 65:12. In the final product, 43% of the lipids were synthetic. In January 1980, Fujiwara and co-workers reported the successful treatment of 10 infants with severe RDS (12). The method of administering the SA was daring. A bolus of no less than 10 ml suspension was instilled into the trachea of preterm infants suffering from severe breathing problems. The large volume probably was needed for an even distribution to all airway branches of the lungs. It was almost as if the neonate was forced to take its first breath once again. The infant was held in different positions so as to facilitate an even distribution of the SA and, as soon as the instillation was finished, i.e., after 20 sec, the lungs were expanded with 100% oxygen and the infant was connected to a respirator. Response to the treatment was dramatic. Grunting when present ceased quickly, blood pressure increased, and peripheral circulation improved. Bowel sounds returned, as did diuresis. Chest radiograms improved faster than they normally would have done without the SA treatment. Blood gas analysis before the SA had been administered showed that the infants were in extremely serious condition, but ventilator pressure could be lowered very soon following the treatment, as could FiO_2, and A-a DO_2 improved rapidly.

There was no mortality because of RDS or the SA treatment, but two infants died, one of sepsis and the other due to complications when operated on for esophageal atresia with tracheo-esophageal fistula. There was one serious problem with the treatment in that no fewer than 9 of the 10 infants receiving SA supplementation developed symptoms and signs of a patent ductus arteriosus (PDA). In fact, the only child not reported as having PDA was the one succumbing at 36 hr from complications of the esophageal atresia operation. The PDA closed spontaneously in four of the infants, but had to be surgically ligated in the other four surviving.

Stimulated by the success of Fujiwara and his co-workers, a clinical trial, similar in design to that of the Japanese, was initiated by Dr Heather Bryan in Toronto, Canada (13). Six infants severely affected by RDS were treated with an intratracheal instillation of 8 ml of an SA suspension containing 25 mg/ml phospholipids, i.e., the total amount of phospholipids administered was 200 mg. The SA was extracted from a calf lung wash. It had a low protein concentration and was sterilized by autoclaving. As judged from the ratio of arterial to alveolar oxygen tension (a/APO_2), there was fast improvement as compared to the values immediately preceding the treatment. The SA substitution was of no benefit to one infant, possibly because the instillation in that instance was technically difficult and incomplete. There was no mortality in the Toronto trial. Four of the infants had normal chest radiograms at 12 weeks. One developed pneumothorax. Another, the infant not responding to the treatment, was diagnosed as suffering from severe bronchopulmonary dysplasia.

A third clinical trial, employing the same principle of treating established RDS with an intratracheal instillation of an SA suspension bolus, was reported by Hallman et al. (14). The SA used was different, however, in that it was not of bovine but of human origin, from amniotic fluid collected at elective cesarean sections at term. Vernix was removed by filtering through gauze, and cell debris by a 10-min centrifugation at low speed. From the supernatant, the SA was isolated with densitogradient centrifugation. The final SA suspension was administered intratracheally via a feeding catheter introduced through the endotracheal tube. The SA was given as a single bolus of 3.5 ml/kg, which corresponded to 60 mg dry SA per kg body weight. Five infants were given SA and compared with others not receiving SA, but otherwise treated similarly and matched for age, birth weight, Apgar score, and severity of RDS. The infants to whom the SA was administered had a milder course of the disease, and FiO_2 as well as ventilator pressure could be lowered faster.

The three clinical trials referred to above have in common that SA, at least partly originating from material naturally synthetized in lungs, was instilled into the trachea as a suspension. Morley et al. (15) took a different approach. They used a totally artificial SA prepared from two synthetic phospholipids, DPPC and unsaturated PG, in a molar ratio of 7:3. They found that when this phospholipid mixture was sprinkled as a dry powder on the water surface of a Wilhelmy balance, the lipids adsorbed very rapidly. Almost instantaneously, they formed a monomolecular film which, when compressed, lowered surface tension to close to zero. The problem previously encountered with the totally artificial SA seemingly had been solved. However, studies on artificially-ventilated premature rabbits did not show that the dry SA gave the impressive and consistent improvement in lung compliance as did a suspension of natural SA (16).

Morley et al. (15) reported the results of treating 22 infants born at 34 weeks or earlier. Using a special device, 25 mg of the dry SA powder was administered. Thirty-three babies, born at the same hospital in the same period of time, served as controls. There was no true randomization, however, and the infants receiving SA and the controls were treated by different physicians. There was not the dramatic effect on blood gases seen in the trials where SA was given as a suspension. Morley has noted lately that the treatment causes a significant reduction in the need for extra oxygen (17). In Morley's first trial (15), there was a conspicuous difference in mortality in that none of the treated babies died, as compared to eight of the controls.

Aside from the high incidence of PDA in Fujiwara's series (12), there have been no negative effects attributable to the administered SA. In the four clinical trials quoted above, there was no fatality among the 43 infants treated with SA. This in itself is quite remarkable, considering that all were born at a gestational age of 34 weeks or less.

A second dose of SA was never administered in the clinical trials quoted, although it seemed clear that the immediate benefits were gradually lost. This is in accord with the observations of Jobe et al. (18), who studied the effect of SA supplementation in preterm lambs. In their experiment, the effect of a tracheal SA instillation lasted only about three hours when the treatment was withheld until serious breathing problems had already developed. However, when the SA was instilled immediately after birth, the effect was more dramatic and of longer duration. This is hardly surprising, since an SA instillation is more likely to be beneficial just prior to the first breath. If deposited as a high concentration bolus into the trachea, the SA can be expected to remain at the air–liquid interfaces during the initial aeration as finer and finer airways open up. This would reduce surface tension and, thus, resistance to aeration; an even distribution of air would be promoted. The SA would reach and outline cylindrical, terminal airways as well as alveoli and offer stability. Under these conditions of smooth, even and stable lung expansion, hyaline membranes might never develop, and SA synthesis should not be disturbed by hypoxia or acidosis. Once hyaline membranes have formed, SA supplementation is less likely to be successful. Then, some airways will be atelectatic and others overexpanded, and an even distribution of the SA supplied is inconceivable. Furthermore, epithelial damage and hyaline membranes already developed will interfere with normal lung function, perhaps partly because of leakage into the airways of proteins with SA-inhibiting effect (19).

In summary, there are reasons to believe that SA supplementation will be more effective if offered before an SA deficiency has had time to cause a disruption of normal lung expansion and architecture. Administration prior to the first breath would be ideal and is presently being tested with a clinical trial at the University of Toronto. Infants at high risk of developing RDS, born at a gestational age of 29 weeks or less, are randomized to receive the treatment or serve as controls. The SA used is prepared by Dr Fred Possmayer of the University of Western Ontario. It is of bovine origin, an extract of calf lung wash with low protein content, autoclaved for sterility. Its phospholipid concentration is 25 mg/ml. The first breath is inhibited manually until the infant has been intubated and the SA instilled into the tracheal tube, 4 ml to infants 28 or 29 weeks and 3 ml to those of still lower gestational age.

Neonatal RDS may have several causes, but SA deficiency certainly would seem to be the most important. Treating with instillation of SA into the airways will be a test case for the concept of SA supplementation. If the treatment is successful, questions raised will be: Can SA supplementation be used as therapy for other respiratory ailments? Are there other conditions with SA deficiency as a dominating problem? There is general agreement that SA deficiency is an important factor in adult RDS, although certainly not the only problem. I expect that very soon we will see papers describing the use of SA as treatment of adult RDS. First, we probably will be reading casuistic reports on how SA supplementation was used as a last desperate resort in moribund patients. Under those conditions, the concept may not have been given a fair chance. The SA should have been supplemented long before its deficiency had seriously harmed the patient.

Recently, Lachmann (20) reported the following experiment. Dogs with virus pneumonia were anesthetized and ventilated with a respirator. The thorax was opened and it could be seen that the lungs collapsed at each end-expiration. Following an SA instillation into the trachea, the lungs were given stability, and blood gases improved. The experiment, shown in a movie, was most convincing.

A few years ago, I reported the following experiment (21). The lung edges of two 27-day rabbit fetuses were photographed as the lungs were expanded with air. Into the trachea of one pair of lungs, SA was instilled. At 27 days, the lungs are severely SA deficient, and the supplementation had a dramatic effect. The lungs expanded better, but a striking difference became apparent, particularly during expiration, in that the cylindrical terminal airways in the treated lungs remained open, whereas in the control lungs they collapsed and air was trapped in distended alveolar sacs. From the law of Laplace, as it applies to a spherical surface, $\Delta P = 2\gamma/r$, and as it applies to a cylindrical surface, $\Delta P = 2\gamma/r$, it is clear that collapse is to be expected in the cylindrical airway provided its radius is less than half that of the spherical alveolar surface. The radius of the cylindrical airway will often be considerably less than half that of the alveolus. We can therefore expect that collapse will not be of the alveolar sac but in the terminal cylindrical airway. Could this give rise to small airway resistance, a part of the breathing problem in asthma? I believe yes, and I would like to point out the effect that drugs used for treating asthma have on the SA system. The β_2-receptor agonists, such as salbutamol or terbutaline, cause a fast release of SA from the cytoplasm of alveolar cells type II into the alveolar space (22, 23). At the same time, the β-receptor agonists reduce the net flow of water from capillaries to the hypophase, the liquid outlining the alveoli (24, 25). This increases the concentration of SA in the hypophase. Glucocorticoids, also of major importance in the treatment of asthma, are well known to accelerate the synthesis of SA in the fetal lung (26). Might it not be that asthma is a condition of relative SA deficiency which becomes so severe during the attack that small cylindrical airways tend to collapse during expiration? Perhaps the acute deficiency could be prevented and the disease kept under control by intermittent prophylactic SA supplementation? In that case, when SA is to be administered into open airways, it probably would be in the form of an aerosol spray rather than as a suspension.

I feel that we are just at the beginning of an era of SA supplementation. I find it surprising that major drug companies are not seriously involved in the development of artificial SA, not containing protein, which can be administered either as a suspension or as an aerosol spray. But the drug companies are not likely to let us know about their early-stage research, so perhaps there is more going on than we realize.

ACKNOWLEDGEMENT

This work was supported Medical Research Council of Canada Grant MT-4497.

REFERENCES

1. Enhorning G, Robertson B: Lung expansion in the premature rabbit fetus after tracheal deposition of surfactant. Pediatrics 50:58, 1972
2. Enhorning G, Grossmann G, Robertson B: Tracheal deposition of surfactant before the first breath. Am Rev Respir Dis 107:921, 1973

3. Enhorning G, Grossmann G, Robertson B: Pharyngeal deposition of surfactant in the premature rabbit fetus. Biol Neonate 22:126, 1973

4. Robertson B, Enhorning G: The alveolar lining of the premature newborn rabbit after pharyngeal deposition of surfactant. Lab Invest 31:54, 1974

5. Enhorning G, Robertson B, Milne E, Wagner R: Radiological evaluation of the premature rabbit neonate after pharyngeal deposition of surfactant. Am J Obstet Gynecol 121:475, 1975

6. Enhorning G, Hill D, Sherwood G, Cutz E, Robertson B, Bryan C: Improved ventilation of prematurely-delivered primates following tracheal deposition of surfactant. Am J Obstet Gynecol 132:529, 1978

7. Adams FH, Enhorning G: Surface properties of lung extracts. I. A dynamic alveolar model. Acta Physiol Scand 68:23, 1966

8. Enhorning G: A pulsating bubble technique for evaluating pulmonary surfactant. J. Appl Physiol 43:198, 1977

9. Robillard E, Alarie Y, Dagenais-Perusse P, Baril E, Guilbeault A: Microaerosol administration of synthetic β-γ-dipalmitoyl-L-α-lecithin in the respiratory distress syndrome: preliminary report. Can Med Assoc J 90:55, 1964

10. Chu J, Clements JA, Cotton EK, Klaus MH, Sweet AY, Tooley WH: Neonatal pulmonary ischemia. I. Clinical and physiological studies. Pediatrics 40:709, 1967

11. Notter RH, Morrow PH: Pulmonary surfactant: A surface chemistry viewpoint. Ann Biomed Engl 3:119, 1975

12. Fujiwara T, Chida S, Watabe Y, Maeta H, Morita T, Abe T: Artificial surfactant therapy in hyaline-membrane disease. Lancet i:55, 1980

13. Smyth JA, Metcalfe IL, Duffty P, Possmayer F, Bryan MH, Enhorning G: Hyaline membrane disease treated with bovine surfactant. Pediatrics 71:913, 1983

14. Hallman M, Merritt TA, Schneider H, Epstein BL, Mannino F, Edwards DK, Gluck L: Isolation of human surfactant from amniotic fluid and a pilot study of its efficacy in respiratory distress syndrome. Pediatrics 71:473, 1983

15. Morley CJ, Miller N, Bangham AD, Davis JA: Dry artificial lung surfactant and its effect on very premature babies. Lancet i:64, 1981

16. Morley C, Robertson B, Lachmann B, Nilsson R, Bangham A, Grossmann G, Miller N: Artificial and natural surfactant. Arch Dis Child 55:758, 1980

17. Morley C: Personal communication

18. Jobe A, Ikegami M, Glatz T, Yoshida Y, Diakomanolis E, Padbury J: Duration and characteristics of treatment of premature lambs with natural surfactant. J Clin Invest 67:370, 1981

19. Ikegami M, Jobe A, Glatz T: Surface activity following natural surfactant treatment in premature lambs. J. Appl Physiol 51:306, 1981

20. Lachmann B: Presentation at 2nd International Symposium on Surfactant Research, Marburg, Germany, September 1983

21. Enhorning G: Photography of peripheral pulmonary airway expansion as affected by surfactant. J Appl Plysiol 42:976, 1977

22. Ekelund L, Burgoyne R, Brymer D, Enhorning G: Pulmonary surfactant release in fetal rabbits as affected by terbutaline and aminophyllin. Scand J Clin Lab Invest 41:237, 1981

23. Oyarzun MJ, Clements JA: Control of lung surfactant by ventilation, adrenergic mediators, and prostaglandins in he rabbit. Am Rev Respir Dis 117:879, 1978

24. Enhorning G, Chamberlain D, Contreras C, Burgoyne R, Robertson B: Isoxsuprine-induced release of pulmonary surfactant in the rabbit fetus. Am J Obstet Gynecol 129:197, 1977

25. Olver RE, Walters DE: The effect of catecholamines on fetal lung liquid secretion. J Physiol (Proceedings) 273(2):58P–59P, December 1977

26. Kotas RV, Avery ME: Accelerated appearance of pulmonary surfactant in the fetal rabbit. J Appl Physiol 30:358, 1971

6. MANAGEMENT OF ASPHYXIA AND INTRACRANIAL HEMORRHAGE IN THE NEWBORN

N.W. Svenningsen

INTRODUCTION

Neonatal asphyxia and intracranial (intracerebral-intraventricular) hemorrhages are associated with both a high risk of neonatal mortality and short-term and long-term morbidity and handicaps (1, 2, 3). In spite of the widespread introduction of continuous intrapartum fetal monitoring and diagnostic techniques like ultrasound screening and computerized tomography uncertainties still remain about the role of birth asphyxia per se as the cause of death or neurodevelopment handicap in a child.

The major still unsolved questions are:
– How do antenatal factors affect the prognosis for the asphyxiated newborn?
– How do the mode of delivery, the procedures in attempting to resuscitate a severely asphyxiated baby, the postasphyxial medical care and nursing influence the outcome after severe neonatal asphyxia?

Since the risk of handicap often cannot be predicted with certainty it is difficult to decide to what extent resuscitative efforts should be applied, i.e. when to start and when to stop resuscitation and intensive care treatment. From clinical materials during the 1970s it is wellknown that the severely asphyxiated infant with inadequate respiration and abnormal muscular and reflex activity after asphyxia eventually may develop apnoic attacks and seizures. The risk of postasphyxial deaths and neurodevelopmental handicaps is considerable in those infants (4, 5, 6, 7).

PATHOPHYSIOLOGY

In recent years a multitude of clinical reports have shown a reduction in mortality from hyaline membrane disease but an increased occurrence of intracranial hemorrhages as a major cause of mortality in very low birth weight (VLBW) infants and of hydrocephalus and neurodevelopmental handicaps in both VLBW infants and larger infants experiencing severe neonatal asphyxia (8, 9, 10). Widespread use of computerized tomography (CT) and ultrasound scanning of the neonatal brain and, latterly, measurements of cerebral blood fow velocity and intracranial pressure have led to revised concepts of the causative mechanisms for intracranial hemorrhage (3, 11, 12, 13, 14).

The relationship of these circulatory changes and lesions to the clinical course and the specific management of asphyxiated neonates are still under debate. The particular vulnerability for intracranial hemorrhage in VLBW preterm infants is mainly related to the immature germinal matrix. Intracranial hemorrhage in those infants is ascribed to overperfusion of the microcirculation in the subependymal cell plate whereas hypoxic damage (periventricular leukomalacia) probably results from impairment in cerebral perfusion in boundary zones of the developing brain (15). In the asphyxiated term infant the vulnerable capillary beds are localized in the margins of infarcted areas in the brain. Loss of autoregulation of the cerebral vascular circulation system is presently considered to be a major pathophysiological factor in both VLBW preterm infants and term infants with severe perinatal asphyxia (13, 16).

The initial response to a period of asphyxia at birth is thought to be a redistribution of blood flow to various organs in order to maintain adequate oxygenation to vital organs. Thus there is initially a rise in the blood flow to the brain, the heart and the adrenal glands but a lowering of blood flow to the kidneys, the gastrointestinal tract and the lungs. Data in support of this initial response in asphyxia have been derived from studies in animal fetuses (17, 18). Several infants born after intrapartum asphyxia diagnosed both by fetal scalp pH and cardiotocography with or without low Apgar scores will survive without evidence of cerebral asphyxial damages. This supports the assumption that a redistribution of blood flow occurs also in the human newborn. It is further supported by lack of central nervous system abnormalities in asphyxiated infants who died because of other postasphyxial dysfunctions, e.g. persistent fetal circulation (19). By this redistribution of blood flow tissue oxygenation can be maintained and prevent the development of brain tissue hypoxia and/or cerebral edema. These protective mechanisms may still be overwhelmed resulting in postnatal cardiogenic shock after intrauterine asphyxia (20, 21). Several studies have confirmed that other organ systems than the brain and the heart may be severely affected by neonatal asphyxia, e.g. the lung with persistent fetal circulation (19), the kidneys with lowered glomerular filtration rate (22), acute tubular necrosis or renal venous thrombosis (23), the liver with dysfunction of glycogen metabolism and the gastrointestinal tract with necrotizing enterocolitis (19).

The major pathophysiological events in light–moderate–severe perinatal asphyxia are schematically summarized in Figure 1. Thus the management of the asphyxiated newborn baby must include not only adequate resuscitation, ventilation and oxygenation, correction of acidosis and of circulatory disturbances but also take into consideration imbalances in brain and other organ functions as well. These may impose additional brain damage by deteriorating the condition of the already compromised baby in the postasphyctic period.

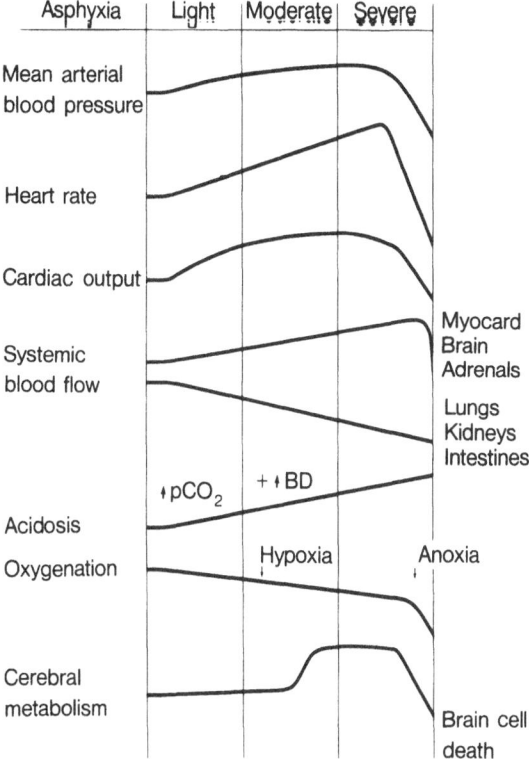

PATHOPHYSIOLOGICAL EVENTS OF PERINATAL ASPHYXIA

Figure 1. Major pathophysiological changes in light to moderate to severe perinatal asphyxia.

GENERAL GUIDELINES

Besides therapeutic interventions the management of neonatal asphyxia must always include the following aspects: 1. *Identification* of the fetus or newborn infant at risk for development of perinatal asphyxia as well as early identification of the actually asphyxiated fetus or newborn baby. 2. *Preventive procedures* applied both before birth and in the postnatal period. 3. *Protective procedures* in order to ameliorate the condition of the asphyxiated baby and to eliminate or at least significantly reduce any prominent brain disturbances, or other organ damages.

Identification

The identification process should start already in the antenatal period of life. Besides clinical obstetrical care antenatal ultrasound scanning and intrapartum fetal heart monitoring and determinations of fetal blood gases (primarily fetal pH) constitute the basic categories of fetal monitoring today. Although they have some limitations these methods of monitoring fetal well-being are well established clinically and can be useful in identification of fetal distress indicating impending asphyxia (24). A fullterm newborn baby with a history of fetal distress from obstetrical monitoring data, low fetus scalp pH, requirement of resuscitation immediately at or shortly after birth (often but not always initial low Apgar scores) and with a change in muscular tone and decreased alertness as a sign of low consciousness level during the first hours of life usually can be identified as an infant with definite fetal and/or neonatal asphyxia.

Preventive procedures

A fully organized and equipped perinatal unit with close fetal and neonatal monitoring (for at least the first 12 hr of postnatal life) is a necessary prerequisite for adequate prevention of asphyxia. It is wellknown that some infants with definite fetal distress may present with Apgar scores in the high range between 7 to 10 but in spite of this eventually develop postnatal signs of asphyxia (5, 25). Therefore postnatal close observation is of paramount importance for both identification, prevention and protection after intrauterine fetal distress.

Protective procedures

For protection against deterioration of the asphyxial process it is vital to stabilize factors, which in imbalance may jeopardize postnatal adaptation processes of cardiovascular functions and metabolism. Function disturbances of cerebral circulatory autoregulation (13) and of cerebral metabolism (26, 27, 28) must be counterbalanced in order to avoid permanent cerebral damage. The primary goal of brain-orientated neonatal intensive care is therefore simply to avoid stressful factors causing imbalances in postnatal and postasphyxial adaption processes (29, 30, 31).

NEUROPATHOPHYSIOLOGICAL BACKGROUND

Asphyxia denotes a state of disrupted placental or pulmonary gas exchange resulting in either total anoxia, but more often hypoxia (partial lack of oxygen), hypercapnea and acidosis. With cessation of gas exchange (placental or pulmonary) neuron reflex-mediated and catecholamine-mediated tachycardia and rising systemic and pulmonary vascular resistance develop. This is followed by a transient rise in arterial systemic blood pressure and a consequent increase of blood flow from peripheral circulation to cerebral circulation. Lowering arterial blood oxygen tension and rising of partial pressure of carbon dioxide will cause dilatation of cerebral circulation. Although these mechanisms are probably compensatory to protect the brain from hypoxia they will be overwhelmed if there is a progressive asphyxia. Increasing acidosis causes cardiovascular collapse with bradycardia and hypotension. Lowering systemic blood pressure causes cerebral ischemia in addition to previous anoxia or hypoxia. Metabolic acidosis through anaerobic metabolism and lactate production will further increase the systemic acidosis by hypercapnea. Hypoxia with acidosis and cardiovascular insufficiency may finally result in profound alterations in the cerebral metabolism. In order to maintain cellular integrity of brain tissue the metabolic demands require endogenous energy from phosphocreatinine and adenosine triphosphate (ATP) and anaerobic glycolysis.

However, the anaerobic metabolism causes accumulation of lactate and thereby further metabolic acidosis. Eventually the high energy phosphate and the glycogen and glucose stores may be depleted. If at this state asphyxia has not been reversed, irreversible cellular brain damage will develop (27, 28, 32).

In this context it is necessary to take into consideration disturbances of cardiovascular function and metabolism which may occur during the recovery period after asphyxia. Partial cerebrovascular underperfusion may persist even after initial resuscitation (13). Partial cerebral edema in damaged areas of the brain may cause water collection and swelling further compromising recovery by an increased intracranial pressure (32). The insufficient autoregulation of cerebrovascular circulation may further jeopardize the cerebral function even by apparently minor events, e.g. during suction of the upper airways, intramuscular painful injections or other procedures in the neonatal care (29, 30, 33).

Persisting disturbances of other organ systems from the initial asphyxial insult also imply risks of additional cerebral damage during the recovery period as earlier described (vide supra, Figure 1). Thus *not only the first hours but the first days after an asphyxial insult in the perinatal period are critical for the long-term neurodevelopmental outcome.* Minute by minute surveillance of the newborn infant in the postasphyxial period and close attention to all details in the recovery phase of asphyxia are of paramount importance.

Neonatal seizures

In newborn infants seizures differ from those seen in older infants and children in two important ways. Firstly the clinical manifestations may be very subtle, probably reflecting the less mature state of the newborn brain both regarding neuro-anatomic and neuro-physiologic development. Secondly in neonatal seizures there is an apparent sparing of vital functions. In contrast to the common overt disturbance of ventilation and circulation seen in older patients such clinical signs may not be apparent in newborn infants (33). However, in recent studies with continuous cerebral function monitoring (CFM according to Prior (34)) for several hours and days we have observed in asphyxiated newborn infants periods over minutes or hours of 'silent seizures' without visible clinical signs of convulsions as illustrated in Figure 2 (35, 36).

In newborn infants an increase of CBF during seizures with or without clinical signs may be deleterious because these infants with a loss of cerebrovascular autoregulation are particularly vulnerable to hemorrhages owing to the immature germinal matrix layer in preterm infants and the vulnerable capillary beds in the margins of an infarcted brain area in asphyxiated preterm and fullterm infants (15, 37, 38). Finally, the cerebral vascular effects from seizures may be accentuated through impaired respiration or apnea during seizures with increase in arterial PCO_2 which is a potent cerebral vasodilatation stimulus (31).

The important questions for management of birth asphyxia are whether the treatment of neonatal seizures is urgent or not and whether preventive measures should be taken?

The well-documented risk of hemorrhagic brain injury during neonatal seizures in addition to the hypoxic-ischemic encephalopathy from asphyxia itself warrants prevention and treatment to avoid seizures. During prolonged seizures the cerebral metabolic activity may increase up to 400% further indicating the importance of urgent and vigorous therapy (39).

Therapeutic procedures

General measures to be taken in order to reach the goal of optimal care of asphyxia as outlined above consequently include organization of a perinatal unit, collaborative preparation and education of the personnel involved underlining the importance of anticipation of fetal or neonatal asphyxia as well as adequate and optimal application of available techniques.

The emergency treatment of the asphyxiated fetus is directed towards elimination of the hypoxic conditions, i.e. immediate delivery of the fetus in order to institute adequate oxygenation and ventilation of the newborn baby. Today the immediate delivery room emergency procedures in cases of asphyxia are well established. In the following emphasis will be put on the postinitial phase of asphyxia, i.e. measurements to be taken in order to establish adequate circulation, to relieve hypoxia and to reduce the metabolic requirements, i.e. to implement a brain-orientated intensive care of the asphyxiated newborn infant.

ANTENATAL MANAGEMENT OF SEVERE ASPHYXIA

Once the fetus or infant with asphyxia has been identified prompt and vigorous

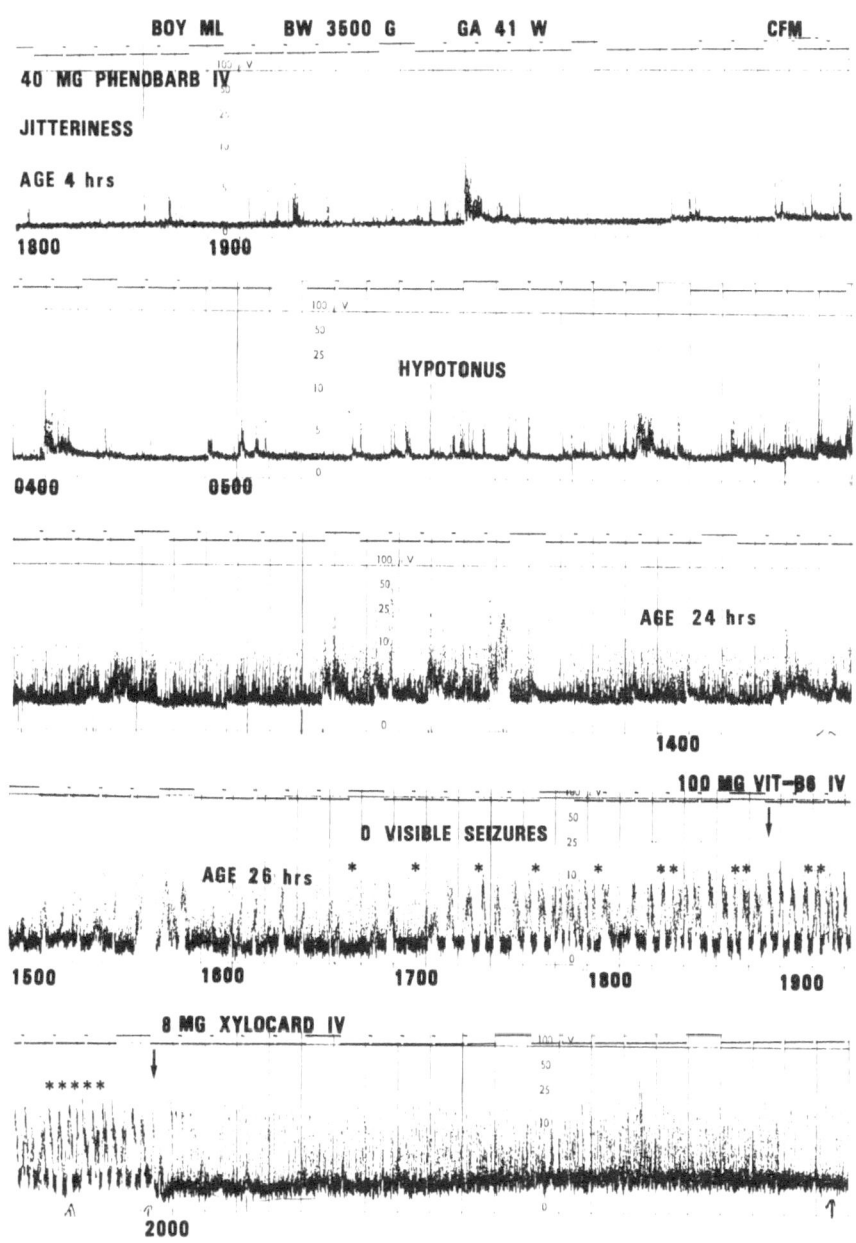

Figure 2. Illustration of 'silent seizures': CFM registration from 3 to 33 hr after severe birth asphyxia with Apgar scores 0(1')–1(5')–4(10'). Initial isoelectric CFM (and EEG). At 4 hr jitteriness treated with 40 mg Phenobarbital i.v. From 15 hr (0500) rising electrographic CFM activity but hypotonus of the baby. At 26 hr (1600) the baby flaccid without visible seizures, but on CFM prolonged electrographic seizures (* *) for several hours. I.v. B6 vitamin had no effect but with i.v. infusion of Lidocain the seizures stopped immediately.

intervention must be initiated in order to avoid a medical catastrophe. The compromised fetus is diagnosed on clinical grounds and by abnormal heart rate and variability on cardiotocography (24) preferably with additional fetal scalp pH determination (40). The decision and timing of obstetrical intervention is crucial for the outcome of antenatal asphyxia. Emergency Cesarean section will usually be needed when deterioration has been documented because vaginal delivery may impose additional risks for birth trauma of an already asphyxiated fetus. Anesthesia techniques applied for the mother also warrant careful considerations. In emergency Cesarean section general anesthesia with combined analgesic agents and muscle relaxants are usually employed (41). Early detection of intrapartum asphyxia and rapid termination of the delivery are the prerequisites for postnatal therapeutic interventions. In conditions of optimal obstetric care postnatal intensive treatment seems justified both from a theoretical point of view and data from pathophysiological animal studies.

Postnatal management

The main principles for management of the severely asphyxiated infant are summarized in Table 1.

The immediate postnatal care of neonatal asphyxia is directed towards rapid cardiopulmonary stabilization, i.e. adequate heart function and respiration either spontaneously or assisted by mask and bag or endotracheal intubation. The main point in the treatment of an infant with severe asphyxia is to relieve cerebral ischemia and to reduce the metabolic cerebral tissue requirements (42).

After initial resuscitation the establishment of adequate monitoring of the baby during the postasphyxial phase is vital. This should include besides clinical assessment of physical and neurological status continuous monitoring of heart function, lung function, systemic blood pressure, and transcutaneous PO_2/PCO_2 as well as repeated measurements of arterial acid–base status, blood gases, electrolytes and glucose. Furthermore, diagnosis of neonatal infection by complete hematologic and microbiological examinations should always be included. Ideally the neurologic assessment should include continuous cerebral function monitoring (ad modum Prior (34, 36)), and EEG with evoked response tests. Structural changes in the brain should be diagnosed by CT scan or ultrasound and cerebrospinal fluid (CSF) analyses. Several of these monitoring techniques can be applied in many neonatal intensive care units with standard clinical equipment. In some specially equipped neonatal intensive care units cerebral blood flow (CBF) with Doppler technique and intracranial pressure can also be estimated. Adequate monitoring is not only important for the initial management but also in evaluation of the progress of the asphyxial process and the effects of therapeutic interventions.

Systemic hypoperfusion as indicated by e.g. inadequate heart rate, abnormal

Table 1. Main features of intensive care management of severely asphyxiated newborn infants.

A. Cardiopulmonary resuscitation	ventilation
	cardiovascular circulation
	arterial blood and tissue oxygenation
B. Brain-oriented protection, i.e. at insufficient ventilation more than 5 min after initial resuscitation	immediately i.v. Phenobarbital (20 mg/kg i.v.) → endotracheal intubation and respirator treatment
sedation prevention/treatment of seizures	Phenobarbital (initial dose 20 mg/kg i.v. maintenance dose 5 mg/kg/day i.v. × 2) Diazepam (1 mg/kg i.v. at seizures) Xylocard: initial dose 2 mg/kg, continuous i.v. infusion (maintenance dose 4–6 mg/kg/hr)
of brain edema and of increased intracranial pressure	restriction of fluid to less than 60 ml/kg/day steroids (Dexamethason 0.25 mg/kg i.v. or betamethasone 2 mg/kg i.v.) respirator treatment with hyperventilation ($PaCO_2$ 25–30 mm HG = 2–3 kPa) osmotic diuresis Furosemide 2 mg/kg i.v. Mannitol 1 mg/kg i.v.
C. Maintenance of body temperature and humidity	
D. Maintenance of systemic blood pressure	continuous mean arterial blood pressure monitoring correction of hypovolemia and blood loss: fresh frozen plasma infusion (10 ml/kg), erythrocytes concentration slow infusions in repeated small volumes (2–5 ml) over several hours (total initial dose of 10 ml/kg)
E. Correction of metabolic disturbances	acid–base balance glucose balance fluid balance electrolyte balance
F. Diagnosis of complication factors, e.g.	persistent (or recurring) fetal pulmonary circulation (PFG) infection renal insufficiency bleeding or coagulation disorders

arterial and venous blood pressure and oliguria, must be diagnosed early and adequately corrected. The etiology of hypoperfusion may be the asphyxia itself or hypovolemia due to bleeding disorders of complicating septic shock. Initial peripheral vasoconstriction may keep the systemic blood pressure within normal range even if hypovolemia is present. In the recovery phase with apparently normalizing acid–base balance there may be sudden peripheral vasodilatation and falling blood pressure. Acidosis may reappear and increase further with release of lactic acid into the circulation. Hypovolemia must be treated preferably with repeated small infusions of 5–10 ml of blood with simultaneous control of blood pressure. The relationship of low CBF with systemic hypotension owing to loss of autoregulation and consequently a high risk for hypoxic-ischemic encephalopathy underlines the importance of blood pressure monitoring. On the other hand rapid volume expansion may be hazardous for cerebral function with risks of cerebral edema or hemorrhages. Volume corrections must be performed slowly with careful monitoring of the circulation and systemic blood pressure.

Close monitoring of body temperature and appropriate adjustment of incubator temperature and humidity is equally important. Correction of acidosis will always be needed once adequate oxygenation and circulation has been established. However, slow infusion of sodium bicarbonate is preferable to rapid infusion which carries a risk of increased serum osmolarity and adverse effects on cerebral blood flow.

Specific brain-orientated management

Protection and treatment of seizures. The occurrence of seizures in postasphyctic encephalopathy must be diagnosed early and treated vigorously. It is equally important to diagnose and treat any hypoglycemia or hypocalcemia or infection causing seizures.

Animal studies have shown that barbiturates may protect fetus and newborns against anoxia, both by prolonged survival time and a reduction and prevention of subsequent cerebral structural damage (43, 44, 45, 46). There are several possible mechanisms whereby barbiturates may have a protective effect, e.g. the sedative effect and the anticonvulsive effect per se, a reduced cerebral metabolic rate of oxygen, the prevention of cerebral edema by membrane stabilization effect and reduction of intracranial hypertension (45, 47, 48, 49, 50). Thus barbiturates can depress the energy demands and also contribute to optimal cerebral energy state during the hypoxia (51). In early animal studies barbiturate administration had a favorable influence on the outcome when given prior to the onset of anoxia but several experimental studies have indicated that barbiturates can ameliorate the effects of brain hypoxia or ischemia even in the phase of resuscitation (43, 45, 46). In later years clinical investigations in both adults and also newborns have indicated a certain protective effect from phenobarbitone treatment (1, 42, 52, 53).

The importance of cerebral edema in the development of posthypoxic encephalopathy or for the long-term prognosis still remains an unresolved problem (54, 55, 56, 57). Cytotoxic edema and focal ischemia may follow hypoxia initially without increase in the intracranial pressure (56, 58). The diagnosis of cerebral edema is often difficult to establish except in cases with bulging fontanell and sutures during the postasphyctic state in a newborn infant. However, other complications like hydrocephalus from intracranial hemorrhage or meningitis must be diagnosed for appropriate treatment (2). If there is clinical evidence of significant increase of intracranial pressure or cerebral edema is suspected in a deteriorating infant measurements should be taken to reduce intracranial pressure, i.e. through fluid restriction, steroid treatment, diuretics, osmotic agents and barbiturates in large doses (see Table 1). In the acute emergency situation controlled hyperventilation aiming at PCO_2 around 3 kPa (= around 25 mm Hg) should be instituted immediately.

Maintenance of adequate blood glucose concentrations during and following asphyxia has been shown to be important since hypoglycemia implies a reduced resistance to anoxia and seizures in newborns (59, 60). Some controversy regarding the optimal level of blood glucose exists as some animal studies have indicated a protective effect by glucose infusions prior to asphyxia (61), while others have found that hyperglycemia did not improve the outcome (62, 63). On the contrary in studies of monkeys elevated glucose concentrations during and after asphyxia were considered to contribute to neurological damage and increase in cerebral edema by surplus lactate production (64). Present recommendations are to administer glucose in an amount sufficient to keep blood glucose within normal levels.

Management of complicating intracranial hemorrhage

Complicating perinatal intracranial hemorrhages during or after asphyxia may occur with either acute dramatic changes in the clinical condition or with no signs or symptoms at all. A sudden deterioration may occur with catastrophic circulatory collapse, hypotension or apnea or with neurological signs such as seizures, abnormal eye movements, hypotonia or a full fontanell. On the other hand sometimes only slight or moderate changes in spontaneous activity or tone or transient bradycardia may be observed. A rapid fall in hemoglobine may indicate intracranial hemorrhage. Today ultrasound scanning or computerized tomography are important noninvasive tools for the diagnosis (2, 3, 8, 11).

Intracranial hemorrhages with large ventricular dilatation and intracerebral bleedings will most often cause neonatal death or neurodevelopmental handicap. However, besides the size of the hemorrhage several other additional factors may be decisive for the long-term outcome, e.g. preceding or intercurrent cerebral hypoxia and ischemia and later additional development of hydrocephalus (5, 10, 65, 66).

Although the exact causative events of intracranial hemorrhages are usually unknown the management is directed towards primarily preventive and protective measures. Thus it has been proposed that liberal use of Cesarean section, for delivery of very immature low birth weight infants in breech presentation or with intrapartal complications, may lower the incidence of such hemorrhages (67, 68). Gentle handling and care both during initial resuscitation and later incubator care are important to minimize sudden changes of oxygen and carbon dioxide tension and arterial blood pressure which may be deleterious because of loss of auto-regulation of cerebral blood flow (29, 31, 69, 70). Furthermore, phenobarbitone treatment in VLBW infants as prevention for periventricular hemorrhage has been recommended although controversial reports have been presented (71, 72). Treatment with fresh-frozen plasma or blood components or drugs with hemostatic effects, e.g. ethamsylate, have also been proposed (73). Decisive evidence through controlled trials of the protective effects from such hemostatic treatments have still not been presented.

In infants with verified intracranial hemorrhage some centers recommend repeated lumbar punctures but contradictory results have been obtained by this approach (74, 75). Surgical treatment with ventriculoperitoneal shunt operation is the method to be preferred in infants with intraventricular hemorrhage developing a progressive hydrocephalus.

The point of no return for such infants is decided by the attitude and philosophy regarding long-term outcome and the capacity (in personnel and technical medical care) in each neonatal unit.

CONCLUSIVE REMARKS

Important new data and knowledge about pathophysiological mechanisms and fetal and neonatal responses to perinatal asphyxia indicate that optimal timing in the management is of prime importance. This is closely interrelated with identification of fetuses and infants at risk in order to prevent or at least ameliorate a progressive asphyxia. In later years animal studies and clinical trials have shown that a certain protective effect can be obtained by optimal intensive care taking into consideration every aspect of circulatory and metabolic events. In the near future improvement in monitoring techniques of cerebral function and cerebral circulation may resolve some of the still unsolved problems in the management of severe asphyxia. At the present time alertness in obstetrical and neonatal surveillance and appropriate application of brain-orientated intensive care, in addition to awareness of preventive procedures, seem to imply a fair possibility to lower mortality rate and incidence of long-term neurodevelopmental handicaps even in some severely asphyxiated newborn infants.

ACKNOWLEDGEMENT

Supported by grants from the Swedish Medical Research Council (grant No 19X-04732) and First of May Flower Annual Campaign for Children's Health.

REFERENCES

1. Volpe JJ: Hypoxic-ischemic encephalopathy: neuropathology and clinical aspects. In: Schaffer AJ, Markowitz M (eds), Neurology of the Newborn. Saunders, Philadelphia, 22:180–238, 1981
2. Flodmark O, Fitz CR, Harwood-Nash DC: Diagnosis and short-term prognosis of intracranial hemorrhage and hypoxic-ischemic brain damage in neonates. J Comput Assist Tomogr 4:775–787, 1980
3. Thorbun RJ, Stewart AL, Hope PL, Lipscomb AP, Reynolds EOR, Pape KE: Prediction of death and major handicap in very preterm infants by brain ultrasound. Lancet i:1119–1121, 1981
4. Brown JK, Cockburn F, Forfar JO: Clinical and chemical correlates in convulsions of the newborn. Lancet i:135–139, 1972
5. Finer NN, Robertsson C-M, Richards RT, Pinnell LE, Petters KL: Hypoxic-ischemic encephalopathy in term neonates: perinatal factors and outcome. J Pediatr 98:112–117, 1981
6. Sarnat HB, Sarnat MS: Neonatal encephalopathy following fetal distress. Arch Neurol 33:696–705, 1975
7. Dykes FD, Lazzara A, Ahmann P, Blumenstein B, Schwartz J, Braun AW: Intraventricular hemorrhage: prospective evaluation of etiopathogenesis. Pediatrics 66:42–49, 1980
8. Fitzhardinge PM, Flodmark O, Fitz CR, Ashby S: The prognostic value of computed tomography as an adjunct to assessment of the term infant with post asphyxial encephalopathy. J Pediatr 99:777–781, 1981
9. Fitzhardinge PM, Pape K, Arstikaitis M, Boyle M, Ashby S, Rowley A: Mechanical ventilation of infants less than 1501 g birth weight: health, growth and neurological sequelae. J Pediatr 88:531–541, 1976
10. Krishnamoorthy KS, Shannon DC, DeLong GR, Todres ID, Davis KR: Neurological sequelae in the survivors of neonatal intraventricular hemorrhage. Pediatrics 64:233–237, 1979
11. Krishnamoorthy KS, Fernandez RA, Momose KJ, DeLong GR, Moylan FMB, Todres ID: Evaluation of neonatal intracranial hemorrhage by computerized tomography. Pediatrics 59:155–172, 1977
12. Schrumpf JS, Sehring S, Killpack S, Brady JP, Hirata T, Mednick JP: Correlation of early neurologic outcome and CT findings in neonatal brain hypoxia and injury. J Comput Assist Tomogr 4:445–450, 1980
13. Lou HC, Lassen NA, Friis-Hansen B: Impaired autoregulation of cerebral blood flow in the distressed newborn infant. J Pediatr 94:118–121, 1979
14. Bada HS, Hajjar W, Chua C, Sumner Ds: Noninvasive diagnosis of neonatal asphyxia and intraventricular hemorrhage by Doppler ultrasound. J Pediatr 95:775–779,1979
15. Wigglesworth JS, Pape KE: Pathophysiology of intracranial hemorrhage in the newborn. J Perinat Med 8:119–128, 1980
16. deCourten GM, Rabinowicz T: Intraventricular hemorrhage in premature infants. Re-appraisal and new hypothesis. Dev Med Child Neurol 23:389–403, 1981
17. Behrman RE, Lees MH, Peterson EN, Delannoy CW, Seeds AE: Fetal circulation in the primate in intrauterine distress. Am J Obstet Gynecol 108:956–969, 1970
18. Kjellmer I, Karlsson K, Olsson T, Rosén KG: Cerebral reactions during intrauterine asphyxia in the sheep. I. Circulation and oxygen consumption in the fetal brain. Pediatr Res 8:50–57, 1974
19. Sexson WR, Sexson SB, Rawson JE, Brann AW: The multisystem involvement of the asphyxiated newborn. Pediatr Res 10:432–435, 1976
20. Lees MH: Perinatal asphyxia and the myocardium. J Pediatr 96:675–678, 1980
21. Cabal LA, Devaskar U, Siassi B, Hodgman JE, Emmanoulidis G: Cardiogenic shock associated with perinatal asphyxia in preterm infants. J Pediatr 96:705–710, 1980
22. Svenningsen NW: Single injection of polyfructosan clearance in normal and asphyxiated neonates. Acta Paed Scand 64:87–95, 1975
23. Dauber IM, Krauss AN, Symchych PS, Auld PAM: Renal failure following perinatal anoxia. J Pediatr 88:851–855, 1976

24. Hon EH, Zanini D, Quilligan EJ: The neonatal value of fetal monitoring. Am J Obstet Gynecol 122:508–519, 1975

25. Nelson KB, Ellenberg JH: Apgar scores as predictors of chronic neurologic disability. Pediatrics 68:36–44, 1981

26. Siesjö BK: In: Brain Energy Metabolism. Wiley, New York, pp 56–100, 1978

27. Vanucci RC, Duffy TE: Cerebral metabolism in newborn dogs during reversible asphyxia. Ann Neurol 1:528–538, 1977

28. Duffy TE, Kohle SJ, Vanucci RC: Carbohyd rate and energy metabolism in perinatel rat brain: relations to survival in anoxia. J Neurochem 24:271–276, 1975

29. Lou HC, Lassen NA, Friis-Hansen B: Is arterial hypertension crucial for the development of cerebral hemorrhage in premature infants? Lancet i:1215–1217, 1979

30. Wimberley PD, Lou HC, Hejl M, Lassen NA, Friis-Hansen B: Hypertensive peaks in the pathogenesis of intraventricular hemorrhage in the newborn. Abolition by phenobarbitone sedation. Acta Paed Scand 71:537–541, 1982

31. Kenny JD, Garcia-Prats JA, Hilliard J-L, Corbet AJS, Rudolph AJ: Hypercarbia at birth: a possible role in the pathogenesis of intraventricular hemorrhage. Pediatrics 62:465–467, 1978

32. Brann AW, Myers RE: Central nervous system findings in the newborn monkey following severe in utero partial asphyxia. Neurology 25:327–338, 1975

33. Perlman JM, Volpe JJ: Seizures in the preterm infant: effects on cerebral blood flow velocity, intracranial pressure and arterial blood pressure. J Pediatr 102:288–293, 1983

34. Prior P: In: Monitoring Cerebral Function. Long-term Recordings of Cerebral Electrical Activity. Biomedical Press, Amsterdam, pp 45–301, 1979

35. Bjerre I, Hellström-Westas L, Rosén I, Svenningsen NW: Cerebral function monitoring following severe asphyxia in infancy. Arch Dis Child 58:997–1002, 1983

36. Hellström-Westas L, Rosén I, Svenningsen NW: Continuous cerebral function monitoring in neonatal intensive care. Crit Care Med (submitted)

37. Lou HC, Friis-Hansen B: Arterial blood pressure elevations during motor activity and epileptic seizures in the newborn. Acta Paed Scand 68:803–806, 1979

38. Minns RA, Brown JK: Intracranial pressure changes associated with childhood seizures. Dev Med Child Neurol 20:561–569, 1978

39. Meldrum BS, Nilsson B: Cerebral blood flow and metabolic rate early and late in prolonged epileptic seizures induced in rats by bicuculline. Brain 99:523–542, 1976

40. Low JA, Karchmar J, Broekhoven L,.McGrath MJ, Parcham SR, Piercy WN: The probability of fetal metabolic acidosis during labor in a population at risk as determined by clinical factors. Am J Obstet Gynecol 141:941–951, 1981

41. Gottschalk W: Anesthesia for emergency obstetrics. In: Aladjem S, Brown AK (eds), Perinatal Intensive Care. Mosby, St Louis, 1977

42. Svenningsen NW, Blennow G, Lindroth M, Gäddlin P-O, Ahlström H: Brain-orientated intensive care treatment in severe neonatal asphyxia. Arch Dis Child 57:176–183, 1982

43. Cockburn F, Daniel SS, Dawes GS, James LS, Myers RE, Niemann W: The effect of pentobarbital anesthesia on resuscitation and brain damage in fetal Rhesus monkeys asphyxiated on delivery. J Pediatr 75:281–291, 1969

44. Goodlin RC, Lloyd D: Use of drugs to protect against fetal asphyxia. Am J Obstet Gynecol 107:227–231, 1970

45. Brann AW, Montalvo JM: Barbiturates and asphyxia, Pediatr Clin North Am 17:851–862, 1970

46. Fisher DE, Patou JB, Behrmann RE: The effect of phenobarbital on asphyxia in the newborn monkey. Pediatr Res 9:181–184, 1975

47. Nilsson L, Siesjö BK: The effect of phenobarbitone anaesthesia on blood flow and oxygen consumption in the rat brain. Acta Anaest Scand Suppl 57:18–24, 1975

48. Gardiner RM: Cerebral blood flow and oxidative metabolism during hypoxia and asphyxia in the newborn calf and lamb. J Physiol 305:357–376, 1980

49. Simeone FA, Frazer GK, Lawner P: Ischemic brain edema: comparative effects of barbiturates and hypothermia. Stroke 10:8–12, 1978

50. Marshall LF, Shapiro HM: Barbiturate control of intracranial hypertension in head injury and other conditions: iatrogenic coma. Acta Neurol Scand Suppl 64:164–172, 1977

51. Vanucci RC, Wolf JW: Oxidative metabolism in fetal rat brain during maternal anesthesia. Anaesthesiology 48:238–244, 1978

52. Brown JK: Infants damaged during birth. Perinatal asphyxia. In: Gairdner DMT (ed), Recent Advances in Pediatrics, 5th ed. Churchill, London, pp 59–88, 1976

53. Finer NN, Robertson CM, Peters KL, Coword JH: Factors affecting outcome in hypoxic-ischemic encephalopathy in term infants. Am J Dis Child 137:21–25, 1983

54. Andersson JM, Belton NR: Water and electrolyte abnormalities in the human brain after severe intrapartum asphyxia. J Neurol Neurosurg Psychiatry 37:514–520, 1974

55. Pryse-Davis MJ, Beard RW: A necropsy study of brain swelling in the newborn with special reference to cerebellar herniation. J Pathol 109:51–55, 1977

56. Fisherman RA: Brain edema. N Engl J Med 293:14–21, 1975

57. Tweed WA, Pash M. Doig G: Cerebrovascular mechanisms in perinatal asphyxia: the role of vasogenic brain edema. Pediatr Res 15:44–46, 1981

58. Selzer ME, Myers RE, Halstein SB: Prolonged partial asphyxia: effects on fetal brain water and electrolytes. Neurology 22:732–736, 1972

59. Vanucci RC, Vannucci SJ: Carbohydrate metabolism in fetal and neonatal rat brain during anoxia and recovery. Am J Physiol 230:1269–1275, 1976

60. Wasterlain CG: Neonatal seizures and brain growth. Neuropädiatrie 9:213–228, 1978

61. Holowach-Thurston H, Hankort RE, Jones EM: Anoxia in mice: reduced glucose in brain with normal or elevated glucose in plasma and increased survival after glucose treatment. Pediatr Res 8:238–243, 1974

62. Dawes GS, Mott JC, Shelley HJ, Stafford A: The prolongation of survival time in asphyxiated immature fetal lambs. J Physiol (London) 168:43–64, 1963

63. Rehncrona S, Rosén I, Siesjö BK: Brain lactic acidosis and ischaemic damage. J Cerebral Blood Flow Metab 1:297–311, 1981

64. Myers RE: Lactic acid accumulation as cause of brain edema and cerebral necrosis resulting from oxygen deprivation. In: Korobkin R, Guilleminoult C (eds), Advances in Perinatal Neurology, Vol 1. Spectrum Publishers, New York, pp 85–114, 1975

65. Mulligan JC, Pointer MJ, Donoghue PA, MacDonald HM, Allen AC, Taylor PM: Neonatal asphyxia. II. Neonatal mortality and long-term sequelae. J Pediatr 96:903–907, 1980

66. Schub JC, Akmann PA, Dykes TD: Prospective long term follow-up of prematures with sub-ependymal/intraventricular hemorrhage. Pediatr Res 15:711–714, 1981

67. Ingemarsson I, Westgren M, Svenningsen NW: Long-term follow-up of preterm infants in breech presentation delivered by cesarean section: a prospective study. Lancet ii:172–176, 1978

68. Greisen G, Petersen MB: Intra-ventricular hemorrhage and method of delivery of very low birth weight infants. J Perinat Med 11:67–73, 1983

69. Perlman JM, McMenahain JB, Volpe JJ: Fluctuating cerebral blood flow velocity in respiratory distress syndrome. N Engl J Med 309:204–209, 1983

70. Danford BA, Miske S, Headley J, Nelson RM: Effect of routine care procedures on trans-cutaneous oxygen in neonates: a quantitative approach. Arch Dis Child 58:20–23, 1983

71. Donn SM, Roloff DW, Goldstein GW: Prevention of intraventricular hemorrhage in preterm infants by phenobarbital. Lancet ii:215–217, 1981

72. Morgan MEI, Massey RF, Cooke RWI: Does phenobarbitone prevent periventricular hemorrhage in very low birth weight babies? Pediatrics 70:186–189, 1982

73. Morgan MEI, Benson JW, Cocke RWI: Ethamsylate reduces the incidence of periventricular haemorrhage in very low birth weight babies. Lancet ii:830–831, 1981

74. Papile LA, Burstein J, Burstein R, Koffler H, Koops BL, Johnson JD: Posthemorrhagic hydro-

cephalus in low birth weight infants: treatment by serial lumbar punctures. J Pediatr 97:273–277, 1980

75. Mantovani JF, Pasternak JF, Mathhew OP, Allan WC, Mills MT, Casper J, Volpe JJ: Failure of daily lumbar punctures to prevent the development of hydrocephalus following intraventricular hemorrhage. J Pediatr 97:278–281, 1980

7. RESPIRATORY MUSCLE FATIGUE IN CHILDREN

JOSEPH MILIC-EMILI

The skeletal muscles are said to be fatigued when they fail to generate the required force. Although there is ample evidence indicating that the inspiratory muscles of humans and animals can be fatigued (for an elegant and comprehensive review, see Ref. 17), the precise nature of this phenomenon has not been established. Skeletal muscle fatigue can be central or peripheral. Peripheral fatigue can be subdivided into failure at the level of transmission (neuromuscular junction and muscle membrane) and failure of the contractile machinery. Although fatigue at the level of the central nervous system or of the neuromuscular junction can occur under certain conditions, fatigue in the contractile machinery appears to be more common (17). Some of the factors predisposing to inspiratory muscle fatigue are listed in Table 1.

Blood flow to the muscles is of crucial importance in relation to their energy supply. Under normal conditions this depends primarily on the intensity of the muscle contraction (during isometric contraction of skeletal muscles perfusion

Table 1. Factors predisposing to inspiratory muscle fatigue. From Roussos (17).

Imbalance of energy supply and demands

(A)	Factors determining energy available
	(a) oxygen content (Hb concentration, O_2 saturation)
	(b) blood flow (cardiac output, distribution of perfusion, ability to increase perfusion)
	(c) stores of substrates (nutrition, previous exercise)
	(d) blood substrate concentration
	(e) ability to extract energy sources
(B)	Factors determining energy demands
	(a) work of breathing ($\dot{V}_E$, V_T, f, T_I/T_{TOT}, resistance, compliance)
	(b) efficiency of respiratory system (breathing through resistance vs hyperventilation, nutrition)
	(c) strength (lung volume, atrophy, prematurity, neuromuscular disease, nutritional status)

Alteration of 'Milieu Interne'

Acidosis, histochemical adaptations, drugs

stops completely when the tension exerted is 70% of maximum) (1, 9) and on the time allowed between each contraction to replenish the energy stores and/or wash out the catabolites. Thus for any intensity of muscle contraction, there will be a critical value of pause duration (relaxation time) below which the blood flow will be insufficient to overcome the debt incurred in the preceding contraction. Thus, in skeletal muscles the blood flow should depend both on tension and timing of contraction.

Although blood flow limitation is known to occur in many skeletal muscles and this has been shown to cause fatigue (17), there is no direct evidence that this does occur also in the human diaphragm or other inspiratory muscles. However, recent studies of Bellemare and Grassino (2, 3) are consistent with the notion that blood flow limitation may be important in determining diaphragmatic fatigue. They have shown that in normal adults there is a fatigue threshold which is reached when the so-called tension–time index of the diaphragm (TTdi) exceeds a critical value. TTdi is the product of T_I/T_{TOT} and $\bar{P}di/Pdi$ max, where T_I/T_{TOT} is the diaphragmatic duty cycle, i.e. the time during which the diaphragm is contracted (T_I), expressed as the ratio of total respiratory period (T_{TOT}); $\bar{P}di$ is the mean pressure developed by the diaphragm during inspiration; and Pdi max is the pressure developed by the diaphragm during a maximum static inspiratory effort performed at functional residual capacity (FRC).

As the duty cycle defines the proportion of time during which the diaphragm is contracted, it also reflects its relative relaxation time. Thus, a T_I/T_{TOT} of 0.5 indicates that the diaphragm is contracted half of the time and relaxed the other half. Similarly, a T_I/T_{TOT} of 1 indicates sustained (tonic) diaphragmatic contraction. For reasons stated above, the timing of diaphragmatic contraction (T_I/T_{TOT}) as well as the tension developed ($\bar{P}di/Pdi$ max) should be important determinants of diaphragmatic blood flow. Thus, the results of Bellemare and Grassino (2, 3) can be interpreted as indicating that, as in other skeletal muscles, diaphragmatic blood flow limitation depends both on timing (duty cycle) and intensity of the diaphragmatic contraction. Once a critical TTdi is reached (about 0.15 for normal adults), the blood flow to the diaphragm is impaired and fatigue ensues. In this connection it should be noted that the oxygen cost of breathing is closely related to the tension–time index of the respiratory muscles (11). Consequently, increasing $\bar{P}di$ may not only cause decreased diaphragmatic blood flow (decreased energy supply) but it also elicits an increased energy demand.

Although other factors than blood flow limitation may play a role in eliciting diaphragmatic fatigue, the results of Bellemare and Grassino (2, 3) provide a useful tool for assessing diaphragmatic fatiguability, as shown in Figure 1. Their plot of T_I/T_{TOT} vs $\bar{P}di/Pdi$ max allows to define the range of fatiguing and nonfatiguing breathing patterns. All patterns which fall above the fatigue threshold will in time lead to respiratory failure due to diaphragmatic fatigue. On the other hand, patterns falling below the fatigue threshold can be sustained indefinitely without the development of diaphragmatic fatigue. Also shown in Figure 1

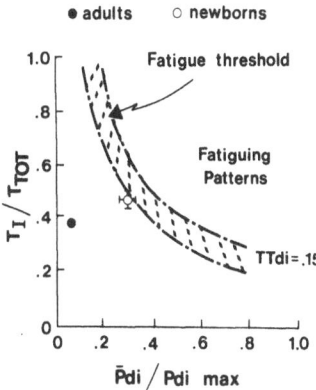

Figure 1. Relationship between T_I/T_{TOT} and P̄di/Pdi max. The hatched area defines the diaphragmatic fatigue threshold, and corresponds to TTdi=0.15. Breathing patterns below the fatiguing threshold can be sustained indefinitely. Filled circle: average value for normal adults during resting breathing. Open circle: estimated value for normal infants. Bars indicate ± 1 SD. After Bellemare and Grassino (2, 3) and Milic-Emili (13).

is the average breathing pattern for normal young subjects breathing room air at rest, T_I/T_{TOT} amounting to about 0.38 and P̄di/Pdi max to 0.07. Since this point lies far from the fatigue threshold, it is evident that normal adults have a large respiratory reserve in terms of fatiguability of the diaphragm.

For infants and children, diaphragmatic fatigue thresholds have not as yet been established. It is most likely, however, that their respiratory reserve is lower than in adults in view of the fact that (a) their resting minute ventilation (corrected for body weight) is greater (8, 14); (b) the maximum inspiratory pressures of which they are capable are smaller (7); and (c) the low compliance of their rib cage (particularly in newborns) promotes its paradoxing during inspiration, rendering the contraction of the diaphragm less effective in terms of generation of negative intrathoracic pressure (14).

In a previous paper (13) which was based largely on theoretical considerations, I have tentatively concluded that normal infants during resting breathing are close to the diaphragmatic fatigue threshold (Figure 1). This notion is consistent with the studies of Bryan and his co-workers (10, 15). Furthermore, I have also suggested that the breathing pattern of infants, which is characterized by high respiratory frequency (f), short duration of inspiration (T_I) and relatively high flows (14), represents a useful adaptive mechanism in the face of decreased respiratory reserve. Indeed, according to my analysis, newborns should not be able to sustain an adequate minute (and alveolar) ventilation by breathing at respiratory frequencies comparable to adults.

In the present paper I will consider the respiratory reserve, in terms of fatiguability of the respiratory muscles, of children. My analysis will be made along the diagram of Bellemare and Grassino (2, 3), as depicted in Figure 1.

For children, only T_I/T_{TOT} data is available. This, according to Gaultier et al. (4), amounts to about 0.45 for 6–10-year old normal children breathing air at rest, as compared to 0.38 in the adults in Figure 1.

Pdi max in normal males amounts to about 190 cm H_2O, and is approximately equally distributed between changes in intrathoracic and gastric pressures, i.e. during the maximum static inspiratory efforts at FRC the pressure developed at the mouth (P_I max) amounts to about 100 cm H_2O ($\approx 50\%$ of Pdi max) (2, 3). To my knowledge, Pdi max for children has not been reported. However P_I max data are available. As shown in Table 2, P_I max in children is smaller than in adults, at least below the age of about 12 years. Assuming that during the maximum static inspiratory efforts of children the changes in intrathoracic pressure represent 50% of Pdi max as in adults, the latter should be decreased in children by the same proportion as Pdi max.

Table 2. Mean values of maximum static inspiratory pressure at FRC ($P_I$max) and of inspiratory duration (T_I) and mouth occlusion pressure ($P_{0.1}$) during resting breathing for children and adults from Refs. 4, 7 and 18. Also shown are estimates of $\bar{P}di/Pdi$ max for children, expressed as % of adult value.

Age (yrs)	P_I max (cmH$_2$O)	P_I max (% adult value)	T_I (s)	$P_{0.1}$ (cmH$_2$O)	$0.5P_{0.1} \times T_I$ (% adult value)	$\bar{P}di/Pdi$ max (% adult value)
6	50	49	1.1	3.0	139	284
8	65	64	1.2	2.4	121	189
10	87	86	1.3	2.0	109	127
Adults	102	100	1.7	1.4	100	100

To my knowledge, $\bar{P}di$ data for children are also not available. A tentative estimate, however, can be made as follows. If the pressure developed by the diaphragm (Pdi) is assumed to increase linearly during inspiration (Pdi=at, where the constant a represents its rate of rise, dPdi/dt, and t is time), it follows that the mean Pdi ($\bar{P}di$) developed during the course of an inspiration (T_I) is equal to $0.5a \times T_I$. Gaultier et al. (4) have provided values of T_I for normal children during resting breathing, as shown in Table 1. In this study they have also measured $P_{0.1}$, that is the mouth occlusion pressure. $P_{0.1}$ is an index of the rate of rise of inspiratory muscle pressure (dP/dt). As shown in Figure 2 and Table 2, this decreases progressively with growth, the adult value of 1.4 cm H_2O being reached at the age of about 14 years.

Table 2 also provides values of $0.5P_{0.1} \times T_I$ of children relative to adults. Assuming that $0.5P_{0.1} \times T_I$ is equivalent to $\bar{P}di$, the latter should increase in children by the same proportion as $0.5P_{0.1} \times T_I$. Furthermore, by dividing this by the corresponding child-to-adult ratio of Pdi max, the child-to-adult ratio of $\bar{P}di/$Pdi max can be estimated (Table 2). Since in adults $\bar{P}di/Pdi$ max during resting breathing amounts to 0.07 (Figure 1), the corresponding values for children can

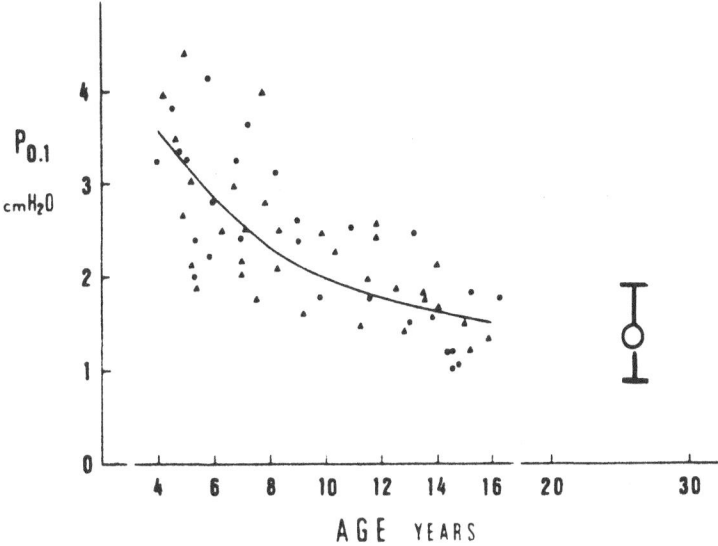

Figure 2. Relationship of $P_{0.1}$ (cmH$_2$O) and age (yrs) in 62 children aged to 4 to 16 yrs. Circles: boys; triangles: girls. From Gaultier et al. (4). Average values ($\pm$ SD) for normal adults of both sexes aged 26 $\pm$7(SD) years from Šorli et al. (18) are also shown.

now be computed. The values of $\bar{P}di/Pdi$ max for children thus derived are plotted in Figure 3 against T_I/T_{TOT} which, in children aged 6–10 years, amounts to about 0.5 (4). It can be seen that in 6-year old children the breathing reserve is relatively small but it approaches the adult value by the age of 10 years. Thus, younger children as well as infants (13) appear to be rather vulnerable to respiratory muscle fatigue when faced with increased respiratory demands (e.g., increased flow resistance, decreased respiratory compliance).

In view of the small breathing reserve of infants (Figure 1) and of younger children (Figure 3), it seems pertinent to consider (a) the therapeutic implica-

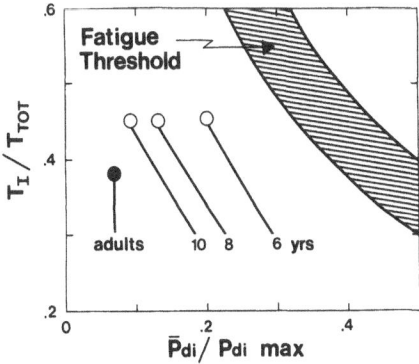

Figure 3. Relationship between T_I/T_{TOT} and $\bar{P}di/Pdi$ max as in Figure 1 but on expanded scale. Filled circle: average value for adults during resting breathing. Open circles: estimated values for children aged 6, 8 and 10 years.

tions, and (b) the strategies of breathing adopted by the patients themselves to prevent ventilatory failure due to respiratory muscle fatigue.

TTdi can be lowered by decreasing T_I/T_{TOT}, decreasing $\bar{P}$di or increasing Pdi max (i.e., diaphragmatic strength). Skeletal muscles, including the respiratory muscles can be trained to increase their strength and endurance (17). The most direct treatment for muscle fatigue is rest which can be achieved by unloading the respiratory muscles (e.g., bronchodilators, correction of pulmonary edema, treatment of respiratory infections) or by instituting artificial ventilation. Prolonged artificial ventilation can, however, lead to atrophy of the respiratory muscles, leading to decreased strength and endurance. The effect of xanthines and catacholamines on the fatigued diaphragm appear to be encouraging in both animals and humans (17). Thus, it is likely that in the near future more therapeutic options will become available to prevent and treat respiratory muscle fatigue.

The patients themselves tend to combat respiratory muscle fatigue by adopting appropriate breathing strategies. For example, infants with hyaline membrane disease exhibit a breathing pattern which is characterized by very short T_I and relatively long expiration. Thus, the T_I/T_{TOT} ratio is decreased and, because of the short T_I, the $\bar{P}$di tends to be minimized. Furthermore, they close or narrow the larynx during expiration which improves gas exchange by preventing collapse of the lung (19). This type of breathing is often associated with an active expiratory effort and a characteristic 'grunting' noise (19). Thus, sick infants appear to respond to respiratory diseases in an appropriate fashion in terms of minimizing TTdi and yet optimizing gas exchange within the lungs. In children and adults faced with respiratory disease, T_I almost invariably decreases tending to minimize $\bar{P}$di, and T_I/T_{TOT} may also decrease, particularly in children (5, 6, 12). Thus, children with respiratory disease by appropriately changing the breathing pattern tend to decrease TTdi, and hence they defend their inspiratory muscles from fatigue. In addition, they may also exhibit alveolar hypoventilation (increased arterial P_{CO_2}) which implies decreased respiratory activity, and hence can also be regarded as a mechanism decreasing $\bar{P}$di. In this connection it should also be noted that the burden on the diaphragm can also be decreased by increasing the activity of the extra-diaphragmatic inspiratory muscles. A most prominent example of this is the 'alternans breathing', characterized by cyclic variations of predominant diaphragmatic or extra-diaphragmatic inspiratory activity (10, 17).

In conclusion, in infants and children aged less than 10 years the respiratory reserve in terms of diaphragmatic fatigue appears to be lower than in adults. In view of the many assumptions on which my analysis was based, it is axiomatic that this conclusion has to be taken with reservations. Nevertheless, it is hoped that this account will stimulate studies of respiratory muscle fatiguability in newborns and children, as this topic appears to be of interest not only from the academic standpoint but also in terms of its clinical implications.

93

REFERENCES

1. Barcroft H, Millan JLE: The blood flow through muscle during sustained contraction. J Physiol (London) 97:17–31, 1939
2. Bellemare F, Grassino A: Effect of pressure and timing of contraction on human diaphragm fatigue. J Appl Physiol (Respirat Environ Exercise Physiol) 53:1190–1195, 1982
3. Bellemare F, Grassino A: Evaluation of human diaphragm fatigue. J Appl Physiol (Respirat Environ Exercise Physiol) 53:1196–1206, 1982
4. Gaultier C, Perret L, Boulé M, Buvry A, Girard F: Occlusion pressure and breathing pattern in healthy children. Respir Physiol 46:71–80, 1981
5. Gaultier C, Perret L, Boulé M, Baculard A, Grimfeld A, Girard F: Occlusion pressure and breathing pattern in children with chronic obstructive pulmonary disease. Bull Eur Physiopath Resp 18:851–862, 1982
6. Gaultier C, Perret L, Boulé M, Tournier G, Girard F: Control of breathing in children with interstitial lung disease. Pediatr Res 16:779–783, 1982
7. Gaultier C, Zinman R: Maximal static pressures in children. Respir Physiol 51:45–61, 1983
8. Jammes Y, Auran Y, Gouvernet J, Delpierre S, Grimaud C: The ventilatory pattern of conscious man according to age and morphology. Bull Eur Physiopath Resp 15:527–540, 1979
9. Humphreys PW, Lind AR: Blood flow through active and inactive muscle of the forearm during isolated hand grip contractions. J Physiol (London) 166:120–135, 1963
10. Lopes JM, Muller NL, Bryan MH, Bryan AC: Synergistic behaviour of inspiratory muscles after diaphragmatic fatigue in the newborn. J Appl Physiol (Respirat Environ Exercise Physiol) 51:547–551, 1981
11. McGregor M, Becklake MR: The relationship of oxygen cost of breathing to respiratory mechanical work and respiratory force. J Clin Invest 40:971–980, 1961
12. Milic-Emili J: Recent advances in clinical assessment of control of breathing. Lung 160:1–17, 1982
13. Milic-Emili J: Respiratory muscle fatigue and its implications in RDS. In: Cosmi EV, Scarpelli EM (eds), Pulmonary Surfactant System. Elsevier, Amsterdam, pp 135–141, 1983
14. Mortola J: Some functional mechanical implications of the structural design of the respiratory system in newborn normals. Am Rev Respir Dis 128:569–572, 1983
15. Muller N, Gulston G, Cade D, Whitton J, Froese AB, Bryan MH, Bryan AC: Diaphragmatic muscle fatigue in the newborn. J Appl Physiol (Respirat Environ Exercise Physiol) 46:688–695, 1979
16. Rochester DF, Bettini G: Diaphragmatic blood flow and energy expenditure in the dog. J Clin Invest 57:661–672, 1976
17. Roussos Ch: The failing ventilatory pump. Lung 160:59–84, 1982
18. Šorli J, Grassino A, Lorange G, Milic-Emili J: Control of breathing in patients with chronic obstructive lung disease. Clin Sci Mol Med 54:295–304, 1978
19. Strang LB: In: Neonatal Respiration. Blackwell, Oxford, pp 205–207, 1977

8. PULMONARY SEQUELAE AFTER ARTIFICIAL VENTILATION

HEATHER BRYAN

INTRODUCTION

Intermittent positive pressure ventilation (IPPV) really began in Denmark in the polio epidemic of 1953 when medical students hand-bagged dozens of patients with bulbar involvement. Lassen's dramatic paper (1) of this reads more like a battle report than a scientific article and converted these tentative steps to the use of IPPV devices as the major method of mechanical support in respiratory failure. This substantially increased the therapeutic range for mechanical ventilators as negative pressure devices were limited in the pressures that they could apply to the lung. It then became possible to treat diffuse parenchymal disease with hypoxic respiratory failure: the two paradigms being infant and adult respiratory distress syndrome (IRDS and ARDS). Now high oxygen concentrations were being forced into lungs with a nonuniform distribution of compliance and created two new problems: pulmonary barotrauma and oxygen toxicity. In a major collaborative study on ARDS it was concluded that over half the patient deaths on conventional mechanical ventilators, were attributed to complications of the ventilator itself; either due to barotrauma or oxygen toxicity (2). A similar situation probably applies to infants with the additional problem of ventilator-induced chronic lung damage, which has no clear counterpart in adult patients.

BAROTRAUMA

It was in IRDS, where the problem was aggravated by pulmonary immaturity, that these dangers first became apparent; indeed clear evidence of ventilator-induced damage in the adult is still ephemeral. In a classic paper Northway (3) described chronic lung lesions which he termed bronchopulmonary dysplasia (BPD). Northway attributed these lesions to oxygen toxicity but the bulk of subsequent evidence is that barotrauma is the major factor in the development of BPD. High-dose oxygen therapy is not directly correlated with the development of BPD (4, 5). On the contrary the severity of BPD is well correlated with peak ventilator pressures (5, 6).

However, it now appears that BPD is simply end stage barotrauma and that the process begins within minutes of instituting mechanical ventilation. Stahlman et al. (7) were the first to show that ventilation of premature lambs led to necrosis and desquamation of bronchiolar epithelium usually accompanied by typical hyaline membranes. They further showed that these lesions were apparent within a few minutes of birth. Adams et al. (8) clearly showed that these lesions only occurred when there was a surfactant deficiency. Schweiler and Robertson (9) further emphasized the role of surface forces as the lesions did not occur during liquid ventilation. They argued that in a surfactant-deficient lung, an air–liquid interface would occur in the terminal airways. Pressure applied to this would distend the terminal airways rather than advancing the interface. The dilatation of the airway would cause disruption and desquamation of the epithelium. While the epithelium of fetal lambs is quite impermeable after mechanical ventilation, the premature lamb develops a very substantial bidirectional protein leak, presumably through the damaged epithelium of the terminal airways (10). This leak can reach astonishing proportions – up to 60 mgm/kg/hr which is virtually a low-pressure pulmonary edema. The shed epithelial debris and the protein leak result in hyaline membranes. The hyaline membranes markedly increase the stiffness of the lung, thus requiring higher ventilator pressures which then compound the damage. Thus hyaline membrane disease is the result of mechanical ventilation, and the infant's own vigorous respiratory efforts may also produce similar damage. If gas exchange can be achieved without creating large intrapulmonary pressure changes then hyaline membrane formation does not occur. Pesenti et al. (11) have had excellent results in premature lambs using apneic oxygenation with extracorporeal carbon dioxide removal and these lungs show no hyaline membrane formation. Similarly, Hamilton et al. (12) in adult surfactant-deficient rabbits, using high-frequency ventilation with a tidal volume of 1–2 ml/kg at 15 Hz did not produce hyaline membranes.

The relationship between the hyaline membranes and the subsequent development of BPD is still speculative. Presumably, either the prolonged use of positive pressure, or the high levels of pressure, cause sufficient tissue damage and an irreversible fibrotic process sets in. Another recently described lesion in BPD is ciliary dyskinesia and abnormal ciliary architecture, both of which resolve with clinical recovery from BPD (13). The cause of these lesions is still unknown, but impairment of the clearance mechanism of the lung must contribute substantially to the development of the lesions in BPD. What role oxygen plays in the development of this condition is debatable and will be discussed separately.

While there is no obvious equivalent to BPD occurring in adults on ventilators for respiratory failure, hyaline membrane formation confined mainly to respiratory bronchioles and alveolar ducts are common to both age groups. Presumably the etiology is the same: when there is alveolar atelectasis, the ventilator overdistends the terminal airways leading to epithelial damage. There is a similar substantial protein leak. In ARDS with its diverse underlying pathological processes, it is much more difficult to unravel what is due to barotrauma and what is due to the underlying pathological process. Macroscopic barotrauma and major air leaks are also not uncommon during IPPV.

Overdistension rather than pressure per se causes the alveolar rupture (14, 15). According to Macklin (16) the highest stresses occur at the alveolar base where the alveolus is tethered to a blood vessel and the commonest site is in alveoli juxtaposed to areas of atelectasis. The air is then forced through the perivascular spaces to the mediastinum and ruptures into the pleural space and may dissect along the great vessels into the neck, or into the retroperitoneal space. The alternative is rupture of a subpleural alveolus directly into the pleural space and if there is an extensive tear this can produce a bronchopleural fistula. These air leaks vary from trivial to life-threatening events, as apart from their effect on gas exchange, they can produce shock and in infants, intraventricular hemorrhage.

Recently we and others (17) have encountered a series of infants with severe necrotic lesions of the tracheal epithelium, distal to the tip of the endotracheal tube causing marked tracheal obstruction. The cause of these lesions is obscure, but they seem to be associated with the new generation of ventilators using high flows to generate 'square wave' patterns. Similar lesions have been reported using 'jet' ventilators. Rapidly advancing technology requires constant vigilance for untoward side effects (18).

OXYGEN TOXICITY

Oxygen has been known to damage the lungs since Lavoisiers' observations in 1787, and this has been repeatedly confirmed in a large, but confusing literature. The difficulty has been that there is a large species variation and great difficulty in ascribing a magnitude to its contribution to the pathophysiology of human lung disease. The problem is that the lung has a limited repertoire of response to lung injury and in the final pathological picture one cannot distinguish between changes due to the underlying pathology, changes due to ventilator barotrauma and changes due to oxygen toxicity. Subjects breathing oxygen for about 20 hr develop both respiratory symptoms and changes in pulmonary function. It is not known whether oxygen toxicity is the result of a high PaO_2 or a high PAO_2. Creating vascular shunts to dissociate these two has led to conflicting results (19, 20, 21). While it is intuitively obvious that oxygen should be more damaging in a diseased lung, the opposite seems to be true. This has been shown in animal models (22) and in two contrasting studies where terminal patients were ventilated with either high or low oxygen. Singer et al. (23), studying patients with cardiopulmonary disease showed no difference in physiological measurements between an FiO_2 of 1.0 or 0.42. Barber (24) studying patients with head injury and presumably minimal lung disease, showed a progressive rise in V_D/V_T and Qs/Qt in his 100% oxygen group. Despite this, the animal evidence of pulmonary injury is so overwhelming that high oxygen concentrations must be regarded as potentially toxic. Some, but not all immature animals are more resistant to oxygen toxicity than mature animals (25). This protection appears to be the result of the neonatal animal's ability to mobilize anti-oxidant enzymes: superoxide dismutase, catalase and glutathione peroxidase. Preliminary reports on the efficacy of exogenous anti-oxidant Vit E have not been substantiated (26). It must be constantly stressed that tissue oxygenation depends on arterial oxygen content and not arterial oxygen tension. With fetal hemoglobin there is little change in content above a PaO_2 of 40 Torr and similarly with adult hemoglobin, little increase above a PaO_2 of 60 Torr. Finally the hemoglobin must be topped up with fresh (not stored) blood transfusions. There is thus nothing one can do to avoid oxygen toxicity; oxygen is necessary and one has to 'grin and bear it', once the strategy for oxygen exchange has been optimized.

ADDENDUM

Ventilatory therapy has been life saving. Our mortality in infants with RDS has decreased dramatically over the past 10 years and today is less than 20%, although higher in the more immature infants. But we must not be complacent, the ventilator in association with supplementary O_2 is a dangerous tool capable of bashing the lung or chemically searing it. Our decrease in mortality has led to a widespread increase in BPD in infants.

The long-term consequences of chronic lung disease are as yet unknown. But data is there suggesting future problems including various degrees of exercise intolerance changing the quality of life, a susceptibility to respiratory infections, and because some of these infants show right heart strain, long-term myocardial function may be adversely affected.

Reynolds showed early that avoiding high-peak ventilation pressures reduced the need for high O_2 concentration and decreased the incidence of BPD. The introduction of CPAP and IMV have further aided our ventilatory techniques. The indications, however, for initiating positive pressure ventilation are much clearer than those for weaning infants from ventilators. In addition, the immature lung in babies <1000 grams may be more susceptible to barotrauma at lower pressures and to O_2 toxicity. Although we have made great strides in reducing mortality with IPPV, we now have major work to do in reducing the sequelae.

REFERENCES

1. Lassen HCA: A preliminary report on the 1952 epidemic of poliomyelitis in Copenhagen. Lancet i:37–41, 1953
2. National Heart Lung and Blood Institute: Extracorporeal support for respiratory insufficiency. Report R.F.P., N.H.L.I. Bethesda, Maryland, p 73, 1979

3. Northway WH Jr, Rosan RC, Porter DY: Pulmonary disease following respiratory therapy of hyaline membrane disease (bronchopulmonary dysplasia). N Engl J Med 276:357–368, 1967
4. Stocks J, Godfrey S: The role of artificial ventilation, oxygen, and CPAP in the pathogenesis of lung damage in neonates: assessment by serial measurements of lung function. Pediatrics 57:352–362, 1976
5. Stocks J, Godfrey S, Reynolds EOR: Airway resistance in infants after various treatments for hyaline membrane disease: special emphasis on prolonged high levels of inspired oxygen. Pediatrics 61:178–183, 1978
6. Reynolds EOR, Taghizadeh A: Improved prognosis of infants mechanically ventilated for hyaline membrane disease. Arch Dis Childh 49:505–515, 1974
7. Stahlman M, Lequire VS, Young WC, Merrill RE, Birmingham RT, Payne GA, Gray J: Pathophysiology of respiratory distress in newborn lambs. Am J Dis Childh 108:375–393, 1964
8. Adams FH, Fujiwara T, Latta H: 'Alveolar' and whole lung phospholipids of premature newborn lambs. Biol Neonate 17:198–218, 1971
9. Schwieler G, Robertson B: Liquid ventilation in immature newborn rabbits. Biol Neonate 29:343–353, 1976
10. Jobe A, Ikegami M, Jacobs H, Jones S, Conaway D: Permeability of premature lamb lungs to protein and the effect of surfactant on that permeability. J Appl Physiol (Respirat Environ Exercise Physiol) 55:169–176, 1983
11. Pesenti A, Kolobow T, Buckhold DK, Pierce JE, Huang H, Chen V: Prevention of hyaline membrane disease in premature lambs by apneic oxygenation and extracorporeal carbon dioxide removal. Intensive Care Med 8:11–17, 1982
12. Hamilton PP, Onayemi A, Smyth JA, Gillan JE, Cutz E, Froese AB, Bryan AC: Comparison of conventional and high-frequency ventilation: oxygenation and lung pathology. J Appl Physiol (Respirat Environ Exercise Physiol) 55:131–138, 1983
13. Lee RMKW, Rossman CM, O'Brodovich H, Forrest JB, Newhouse M: Bronchopulmonary dysplasia: ciliary motility and ultrastructure. Am Rev Resp Dis 129:190–193, 1984
14. Day R, Goodfellow AM, Apgar V, Beck GJ: Pressure–time relations in the safe correction of atelectasis in animal lungs. Pediatrics 10:593–602, 1952
15. Caldwell EJ, Powell RD Jr, Mullooly JP: Interstitial emphysema: a study of physiologic factors involved in experimental induction of the lesion. Am Rev Resp Dis 102:516–525, 1970
16. Macklin CC: The site of air leakage from lung alveoli into the interstitial tissue during overinflation in the cat. Verk Anat 85:78–82, 1938
17. Metlay LA, MacPherson TA, Doshi N, Milley JR: A new iatrogenic lesion in newborns requiring assisted ventilation. N Engl J Med 309:111–112, 1983
18. Silverman WA: The lesion of retrolental fibroplasia. Sci Am 236:100–107, 1977
19. Winter PM, Gupta RK, Michaliski AH, Lanphier EH: Modification of hyperbaric oxygen toxicity by experimental venous admixture. J Appl Physiol 23:954–963, 1967
20. Miller WW, Waldhausen JA, Rashkind WJ: Comparison of oxygen poisoning of the lung in cyanotic and acyanotic dogs. N Engl J Med 282:943–947, 1970
21. Ashbaugh DG: Oxygen toxicity in normal and hypoxemic dogs. J Appl Physiol 31:664–668, 1972
22. Smith G, Winter PM, Wheelis RF: Delayed rate of development of pulmonary oxygen toxicity following oleic acid induced lung damage. Br J Anaesth 45:641, 1973
23. Singer MM, Wright F, Stanley LK, Roe BB, Hamilton WK: Oxygen toxicity in man: a prospective study in patients after open heart surgery. N Engl J Med 283:1473–1478, 1970
24. Barber RE, Lee J, Hamilton WK: Oxygen toxicity in man: a prospective study in patients with irreversible brain damage. N Engl J Med 283:1478–1484, 1970
25. Frank L, Bucher JR, Roberts RJ: Oxygen toxicity in neonatal and adult animals of various species. J Appl Physiol 45:699–704, 1978
26. McMillan DD, Boyd GN: The role of antioxidants and diet in the prevention or treatment of oxygen-induced lung microvascular injury. Ann NY Acad Sci 384:535–543, 1982

9. HIGH-FREQUENCY VENTILATION

A. CHARLES BRYAN

INTRODUCTION

High-frequency ventilation (HFV) is a difficult subject to deal with because we still lack a definition of high frequency. Basically HFV comes in three flavors: high-frequency positive pressure ventilation (HFPPV) introduced by Jonzon et al. (1); high-frequency jet ventilation (HFJV) introduced by Klain et al. (2); and high-frequency oscillation (HFO) introduced by Lunkenheimer et al. (3). The definition of high frequency depends on the system: HFPPV generally operates at 60+/min, HFJV at 150+/min and HFO at 900+/min. They can all achieve effective gas exchange in the normal lung. There are, as yet, no good comparative studies between the systems, nor any convincing evidence that any of them are superior to conventional mechanical ventilation (CMV) in diffuse parenchymal lung disease with hypoxia in humans. Despite this there are compelling theoretical reasons to suspect that HFV may be superior to CMV in this group of diseases. CMV creates large phasic volume distensions in sick lungs which have a non-uniform distribution of compliance, inevitably creating local overdistension. This can, at the macroscopic level, lead to air leaks (pneumothorax, etc.) and at the microscopic level cause hyaline membrane formation. Therefore, a mode of ventilation which reduces the magnitude of the volume distension might reduce the degree of barotrauma.

Following this logic we have used HFV at 15 Hz with a tidal volume less than the volume of the dead space, about 1–2 ml/kg. In conventional physiology there should be no alveolar ventilation (V_A) if the tidal volume (V_T) is less than the dead space volume (V_D). The standard equation:
$$V_A = (V_T - V_D)f,$$
however, breaks down at high frequencies. Henderson et al. (4) and Briscoe et al. (5) both recognized that the dead space volume could be substantially smaller than the volume of the conducting airways.

Lunkenheimer et al. (3) were the first to unequivocally demonstrate that excellent gas exchange could be achieved in dogs with very small tidal volumes and frequencies up to 40 Hz. This remarkable experiment probably did not get the attention it deserved because although gas exchange was excellent, the animals developed a progressive metabolic acidosis, which in retrospect had nothing to do with the high frequency per se, but due to a high mean airway pressure (P_{aw}) reducing venous return and cardiac output. Bohn et al. (6) subsequently showed that excellent gas exchange could be achieved at 15 Hz if the P_{aw} was not too high.

MECHANISM

of the conventional gas transport equations cannot explain HFV, novel mechanisms have to be sought, and a variety of mechanisms have been proposed. Simple convection can ventilate units with a short path length and hence a small local dead space. Asymmetric velocity profiles that occur at bifurcations will lead to deeper penetration than if the flow had been uniform. Finally superimposition of convection on a diffusive process (Taylor dispersion) can substantially facilitate diffusion. Fredberg in the first systematic attempt to explain gas exchange during HFV based his argument on Taylor dispersion (7). However, this analysis would make gas exchange vary directly with velocity ($V_T \times f$) whereas several groups have now shown that it is closer to $V_T^2 \times f$. Whatever the mechanism it is important to note that the distribution of ventilation within the lung will not be the same with the two modes of ventilation. On CMV the tidal volume is distributed in accordance with the regional time constants ($R \times C$), inertia having little influence. On HFV the volume is small so regional compliance is of little importance, but accelerations are high so inertial forces (I) become important, so distribution will be predominantly determined by $R \times I$. This may have a profound effect on lung disease which is often characterized by a nonuniform distribution of compliance.

HIGH-FREQUENCY TACTICS

Entirely different tactics have to be used with HFV. The advantage of CMV is that high pressures are used which will exceed the opening pressures of closed units and hence recruit lung volume. The disadvantage is that usually the end expiratory pressure is below 'closing pressure' resulting in derecruitment. Further, the constant ripping open of closed units appears to be the major cause of epithelial injury and hyaline membrane formation. During HFV, as relatively small volumes are used, relatively small pressures are generated, which may not exceed opening pressure. This situation is quite dangerous as the rapid inflation and deflation of terminal airways is sufficient to produce epithelial injury without much benefit to oxygen exchange.

Several tactical maneuvers have been attempted. HFV can be superimposed on low-rate CMV. Our preferred strategy is to 'sigh' the lung slowly to 30–40 cm of water to exceed opening pressure and then drop the pressure to a level exceeding closing pressure, as theoretically this would maintain the recruited volume (8). This can work extremely well. In a group of adult rabbits rendered surfactant deficient by repeated lung lavage, CMV and HFV were compared. After lavage, both groups were 'sighed' slowly to 30 cm H_2O. The HFV group was maintained on 100% O_2 at 15 Hz with a tidal volume of 1–2 ml/kg at a P_{aw} of 15 cm H_2O. The CMV group was also on 100% O_2 at the same P_{aw}; peak pressures and rate were adjusted to maintain normocarbia and PEEP added to bring P_{aw} to 15 cm H_2O. From Figure 1, it is clear that oxygenation is much superior on HFV. Further, on CMV there was a progressive decrease in compliance and at autopsy the lungs showed extensive hyaline membranes (Figure 2). In contrast on HFV there were no significant changes in compliance and no hyaline membranes (9).

The practical problem is that there are ranges of both opening and closing pressures in more complicated disease models. Thus, in the preterm lamb the upper lobes open satisfactorily at 40 cm H_2O, but the lower lobes often remain atelectatic. Using higher opening pressures risks a pneumothorax in the upper lobes. Similar problems exist with a range of closing pressure: operating above the highest closing pressure may be too high for units with a low closing pressure.

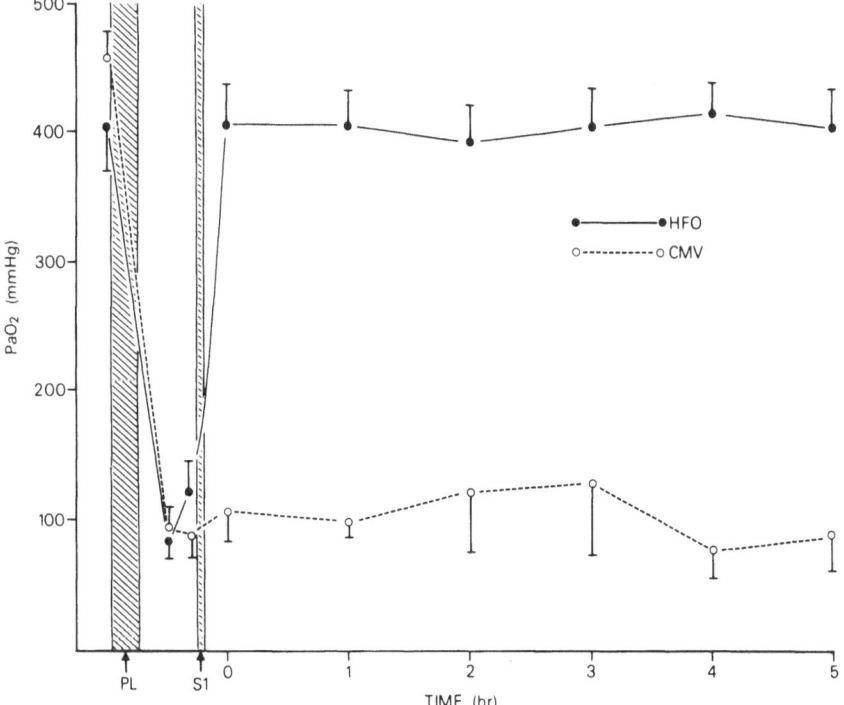

Figure 1. Plot of arterial PO_2 (PaO_2) vs time for 5 experiments. Values appearing immediately before and after wide cross-hatched area represent control values before and after pulmonary lavage. Values appearing before and after narrow cross-hatched area represent pre-SI and post-SI values. Vertical bars denote SE.

104

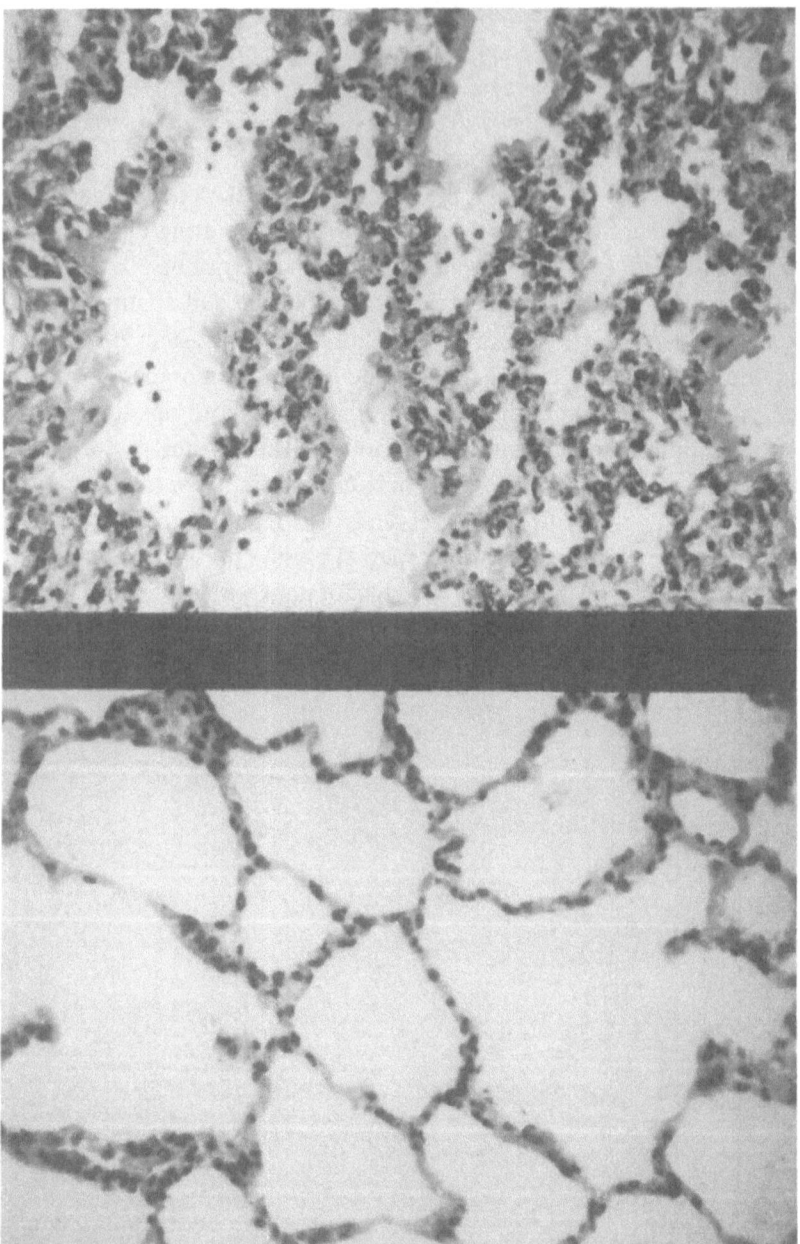

Figure 2. Sections of uninflated lung fixed by immersion in Bouins fixative. Top: diffuse hyaline membrane formation in the uninflated lung of an animal treated with CMV. (H & E stain, ×50). Arrows indicate hyaline membranes. Bottom: appearance of uninflated lung of an animal treated with HFV. There are no hyaline membranes visible (H & E stain, ×50).

CONCLUSIONS

A clear role for HFV has not yet emerged. If the problem is CO_2 elimination (e.g. neuromuscular disease) HFV is excellent – but so are conventional ventilators. The real clinical challenges are acute parenchymal disease with hypoxia: the two paradigms being infant and adult respiratory distress syndromes. There is no doubt that CMV complicates both these conditions with macroscopic and microscopic barotrauma. There is no doubt that theoretically, and in some animal models, HFV can avoid this. But at this time there is no entirely convincing proof of superiority of HFV over CMV. HFV has a few special applications. It is useful in bronchopleural fistula as the fistula constitutes a highly compliant region. It has proved useful in reducing motion in a surgical field (particularly vascular neurosurgery). However, it still remains a research tool, if for no other reason than there is no entirely safe HFV device available.

REFERENCES

1. Jonzon A, Obert PA, Sedin G, Sjostrand U: High frequency positive pressure ventilation by endotracheal insufflation. Acta Anaesth Scand Suppl 43:1, 1971
2. Klain M, Smith RB: High frequency percutaneous jet ventilation. Crit Care Med 5:280–287, 1977
3. Lunkenheimer PP, Frank I, Issing H, Keller H, Dickhut HH: Intrapulmonaler Gaswechsel unter simulierter Apnoe durch transtrachealen periodischen intrathorakalen Druckwechsel. Anaesthesist 22:232–237, 1972
4. Henderson YH, Chillingworth FP, Whitney JL: The respiratory dead space. Am J Physiol 38:1–19, 1915
5. Briscoe WA, Forster RE, Comroe JH: Alveolar ventilation at very low tidal volumes. J Appl Physiol 7:27–30, 1954
6. Bohn DJ, Miyasaka K, Marchak BE, Thompson WK, Froese AB, Bryan AC: Ventilation by high frequency oscillation. J Appl Physiol (Respirat Environ Exercise Physiol) 48:710–716, 1980
7. Fredberg JJ: Augmented diffusion in airways can support gas exchange. J Appl Physiol (Respirat Environ Exercise Physiol) 49:232–238, 1980
8. Kolton M, Cattran CB, Kent G, Volgyesi G, Froese A, Bryan AC: Oxygenation by high frequency ventilation compared to conventional mechanical ventilation. Anesth Analg 61:323–332, 1982
9. Hamilton PP, Onayemi A, Smyth JA, Gillan JE, Cutz E, Froese AB, Bryan AC: Comparison of conventional & high frequency ventilation: oxygenation and lung pathology. J Appl Physiol (Respirat Environ Exercise Physiol) 55, 1983

10. RECURRENT APNEA IN NEWBORN INFANTS

A. OKKEN

CLINICAL DEFINITION OF APNEA

Apnea (Greek; a-pnoia) which means no breath, is a common problem in neonatal intensive care. Usually apnea is defined as the cessation of breathing during a certain period of time. In newborn infants the duration of apnea however varies with the patterns of breathing that range from regular breathing without apnea to extremely irregular breathing with prolonged apneic episodes. Several patterns of breathing are found in newborn infants. Regular breathing with almost equal breath-to-breath intervals and amplitudes (depth of breath) is common in mature newborn infants especially during non-REM (quiet) sleep. Irregular breathing with marked variability in breath-to-breath intervals and amplitudes, in mature newborn infants usually observed during REM (active) sleep, is common in preterm infants. Periodic breathing, defined by cessation of breathing for 3 to 10 seconds occurring at regular intervals alternating with bursts of breahing activity is seen in both mature and preterm newborn infants at sleep (1). The pattern of breathing of preterm infants is mostly irregular and periodic. With increasing gestational age the pattern of breathing becomes more regular and less periodic.

Generally apnea of less than 6 to 9 seconds is considered the be normal in newborn infants (2). Prolonged apnea greater than 15 to 20 seconds however is considered to be potentially harmful because this condition is frequently associated with bradycardia, cyanosis, pallor and hypotonia. In neonatal intensive care the cessation of breathing for more than 15 to 20 seconds is commonly referred to as apnea. It should be emphasized that this is an operational definition used in neonatal intensive care. In sleep studies for instance apnea of a much shorter duration is considered to be significant.

ORIGIN OF APNEA

Apnea in newborn infants may be of central, obstructive or mixed origin. Central apnea originates in the respiratory center in the brain stem. Clinically this type of apnea is usually defined by the complete absence of breathing movements, resulting from the inhibition of respiratory muscle activity. Obstructive apnea originates in the upper airway. This type of apnea is the result of closure of the airway at the level of pharynx and/or larynx through a variety of conditions including relaxation of muscles and head and neck flexion. Clinically obstructive apnea is not detected as easily as central apnea since it requires the measurement of airflow at nose and mouth. Mixed apnea is a type of apnea in which both central and obstructive apnea are observed. Usually mixed apnea starts with central apnea followed by obstructive apnea. Since upper airway obstruction is often associated with inspiratory breathing efforts, obstructive apnea may not be detected unless air flow at nose and mouth is measured. Consequently monitoring systems sensitive to breathing movements may fail to detect obstructive apnea. Alternatively apnea has been redefined as 'absence of air flow at nose and mouth' (3) instead of 'absence of breathing movements'. In term infants all three types of apnea are observed.

In preterm infants, apnea was thought to be predominantly of central origin. Recent reports (4) however indicate that obstructive and mixed apnea may comprise 50 to 90% of apneic episodes in some preterm infants.

APNEA AND BRADYCARDIA

Apneic episodes lasting 15 to 20 seconds or longer are complicated by bradycardia. In preterm infants this is observed more frequently than in fullterm infants (5, 6). In some infants the fall in the heart rate occurs very early in the apneic episode. In these infants bradycardia my result primarily from vagal influences on cardiorespiratory control. Bradycardia not clearly associated with prolonged apnea has been referred to as 'nonapnea-associated bradycardia'. 'Nonapnea-associated bradycardia' however is always associated with changes in respiratory pattern (7). This type of bradycardia has been observed during short episodes of respiratory abnormalities at sleep associated with body movements, during minor changes in respiratory pattern and during prolonged apnea if the apnea alarm failed. Obviously the last occasion should not be considered a 'nonapnea-associated breathing' from a pathophysiological point of view.

CONDITIONS ASSOCIATED WITH APNEA

Conditions associated with an increased incidence of apnea are listed in Table 1. Several of these conditions are related to major clinical problems in the neonatal period. However even without these problems newborn infants may have recurrent apneic episodes. This especially relates to apnea of prematurity and apnea during sleep.

Table 1. Conditions associated with recurrent apnea in newborn infants.

Condition	Major clinical problems
Prematurity	Infants less than 1.5 kg birth weight and less than 32–33 weeks gestational age
Sleep	Predominantly REM (active) sleep
Disorders of the central nervous system	Asphyxia and edema, intracranial hemorrhage, seizures and malformations
Infection	Neonatal sepsis/meningitis, necrotizing enterocolitis
Patent ductus arteriosus	Increased incidence of apnea with increasing left-to-right shunt and pulmonary edema
Respiratory distress syndrome	Increased incidence of apnea possibly related to stiff lungs and chest wall distortion
Metabolic disorders	Hypoglycemia, hypocalcemia, hypo- and hypernatremia, hyperammonemia
Thermal instability	Apneic episodes associated with rises and falls in the environment (incubator) temperature
Drugs	Drugs given to or taken by the mother

Prematurity

Recurrent apnea occurs predominantly in preterm infants of less than 1.5 kg body weight (6). The incidence increases dramatically with decreasing gestational age (5, 6) as does periodic breathing. If no abnormalities seem to exist recurrent apnea in these infants is designated 'idiopathic apnea of prematurity'. The pathophysiology of apnea of prematurity is still poorly understood. The respiratory control is very preterm infants differs from that in fullterm infants. During periodic breathing, which occurs frequently in preterm infants the respiratory control system seems to be depressed as may be concluded from the shift in the CO_2 response curve to the right. In addition the ventilatory response to CO_2 is less in very preterm infants (8). Mild hypoxia may induce periodic breathing in preterm infants (9) resulting in an increased incidence in apnea. In both fullterm and preterm infants the ventilatory response to hypoxia is different from that in the adult. In newborn infants hypoxia results in a very short increase in ventilation followed by a decrease resulting in prolonged hypoxia (10). In preterm infants hypoxia also decreases the ventilatory response to CO_2. It is suggested that this paradoxic response in newborn infants has a central origin (11).

Sleep

A major part of apneas occurs predominantly durig REM (active) sleep and indeterminate (transitional) sleep in both preterm and term infants. Although several mechanisms have been proposed, the high incidence of apnea during REM sleep is not yet fully understood. Evidence has been found that behavioral activity during REM sleep decreases the ventilatory response to hypoxia (11). In this respect the decreases PaO_2 observed in newborn infants during REM sleep (12, 13) needs further exploration. Furthermore paradoxical chest wall movements (inward movement during inspiration) during REM sleep are suggested to exhibit the intercostal to phrenic inhibitory reflex (14). In addition the more compliant chest wall in REM sleep might affect lung and chest wall mechanisms (15) resulting in respiratory periodicity and diaphragmatic fatigue (16).

Disorders of the central nervous system

Intracranial hemorrhage is a common cause of recurrent apnea of central origin in the neonatal period. If apnea occurs in the immediate neonatal period edema and/or intracranial hemorrhage may be the result of anoxia before or during birth. In the absence of other diseases this may be the only cause of apnea. Apneas associated with seizures are much less frequent, apneas related to malformations are rare. Presently a major part of abnormalities of the central nervous system can be diagnosed by ultrasound techniques.

Infection

Sepsis/meningitis and necrotizing enterocolitis may cause apnea of central origin. It is suggested that pneumonia may cause apnea through vagal reflex activity and hypoxemia (11).

Patent ductus arteriosus

Patent ductus arteriosus is one of the major problems in preterm infants. Studies reveal that the incidence of apnea increases with increasing left-to-right shunt and pulmonary edema, associated with an increase in $PaCO_2$ and a decrease in PaO_2. After closure of the ductus the incidence of apnea decreases (17).

Respiratory distress syndrome

Recurrent apnea is present in infants with the respiratory distress syndrome. Possible pathophysiological mechanisms being exhaustion of the respiratory muscles and distortion of the chest wall. It should be realized, however, that patent ductus arteriosus is also a common complication in this disease. It has also been shown that the total duration of apneas greater than 5 sec is significant less in infants with RDS during the first day of life. This phenomenon could not be demonstrated on the third and seventh day of life (18).

Metabolic disorders

Apnea associated with metabolic disorders such as hypoglycemia, hyper- and hyponatremia and hyperammonemia is probably of central origin. These apneas may be eliminated by measures that correct the metabolic abnormality. Apnea associated with hypocalcemia may be an incidental finding (18).

Thermal instability

Increased environmental (incubator) temperature is associated with apnea. Apneic episodes also are frequently preceded by changes in environmental temperature (5, 19). Increased environmental temperature probably acts through inhibition of the respiratory center. Decrease of environmental temperature to the lower neutral temperature range mostly will diminish apnea due to a too hot environment.

Drugs

Several drugs given to or taken by the mother may depress the infant's respiratory activity. Careful examination of the patient history may be necessary. Since most drugs are eliminated slowly by newborn infants their action may last for several days.

MONITORING OF APNEA

Several types of respiration monitors are presently available. Generally the techiques for monitoring respiration either exist of systems that sense exchange of air in or outside the airways (direct method) or detect breathing movements or changes in physical properties in the lungs related to breathing (indirect methods). Direct methods include the measurement of temperature changes between in- and expiratory air (thermistor probes), CO_2 changes during expiration (capnograph), changes in airway pressure (pressure transducer) and detection of air flow (pneumotachograph). Indirect methods of monitoring respiration include the detection of changes in pulmonary air and blood volume (impedance pneumograph), detection of body movements related to breathing (air mattress, capacitive mattress and pressure transducer mattress) and the measurement of changes in circumference of chest wall and/or abdomen during breathing (mercury in rubber strain gauges, air-filled tubing pneumograph). Since direct methods will detect changes in air movement in or outside the airways irrespective of their origin, central and obstructive apnea can be reliably monitored using such methods. Because obstructive apnea may occur in combination with active breathing movements indirect methods may fail to detect obstructive and or mixed apnea although central apnea generally will be detected. Unfortunately respiration monitors most widely used in neonatal intensive care are based on indirect methods (impedance pneumograph, several types of mattresses). Although these monitors are easy to operate and reliable to detect central apnea, their disadvantage in monitoring obstructive and/or mixed apnea is obvious. Actually the incidence of obstructive and/or mixed apnea in neonatal intensive care until now may have been underestimated using these types of monitors. Nevertheless respiration monitors although not ideal have been considerably helpful in neonatal intensive care. The combination of respiration monitoring and heart rate monitoring in neonatal intensive care has several advantages. One of the most important advantages being the detection of bradycardia in those infants in which respiration monitors fail to detect (obstructive and/or mixed) prolonged apneic episodes.

TREATMENT OF APNEA

Treatment of apnea should be based on the cause of apnea. Because several conditions are associated with apnea in the neonatal period (Table 1) there is not a single treatment of apnea. In newborn infants with apnea a careful examination as to possible causes should be performed. Depending on the clinical status of the infant this may include a metabolic evaluation and septic workup. In general diagnostic procedures as to possible causes of apnea are started when infants with apneic episodes require vigorous stimulation or mask and bag ventilation to reinitiate normal breathing. Suggested steps in the diagnosis of possible causes of apnea in the neonatal period are listed in Table 2. Causes should be treated. If no possible cause of apnea can be detected in premature infants 'idiopathic apnea of prematurity' should be considered.

Table 2. Suggested steps in the diagnosis of possible causes of apnea in the neonatal period.

- Check environmental temperature and/or incubator temperature
- Examine the infant carefully. Are apneas of central or obstructive origin? In infants with respiratory distress syndrome is there evidence of patent ductus arteriosus? Check for hypoxemia.
- Consider the possibility of intracranial hemorrhage
- Check for metabolic disorders (including blood gas analysis) and infection as listed in Table 1
- Check the infants medical history, is there evidence of asphyxia at birth
- Check for drugs administered to the mother or the infant

Several sensory stimuli have been shown to decrease apnea in preterm infants. These include cutaneous proprioceptive or vestibular stimulation via nurses, parents or the use of an oscillating water bed (20). A low continuous positive airway pressure (3–5 cm H_2O) has also been shown to decrease the incidence of apnea in preterm infants, its mode of action however is still unclear (21).

Xanthine drugs (theophylline and caffeine) (22) presently have become very popular in the treatment of apnea in premature infants. The recommended dose of theophylline is 5 mg/kg body weight loading dose followed by 1 mg/kg body weight every 8 hr to achieve a therapeutic plasma level of 10 μg/ml. Despite accumulating studies the precise mode of action of these drugs is not yet resolved. At the currently recommended dose the ventilatory response to CO_2 seems to be unaffected. Increased levels of 3,5 cyclic AMP may play a role in increased respiratory drive in these infants.

In some infants with apnea who do not respond to treatment repeated mask and bag ventilation may be necessary. This procedure however is not without risks including hyperoxia (23). In such infants artificial ventilation should be considered.

REFERENCES

1. Hoppenbrouwers T, Hodgman JE, Harper RM, Hofman E, Sterman MB, Mc Ginty DJ: Polygraphic studies of normal infants during the first six months of life. III. Incidence of apnea and periodic breathing. Pediatrics 60:418, 1977
2. Hoppenbrouwers T, Hodgman JE, Kazuko Arakawa, Harper R, Sterman B: Respiration during the first six months of life in normal infants. III. Computer identification of breathing pauses. Pediatr Res 14:1230, 1980
3. Guilleminault C, Periata R, Souquet M, Dement WC: Apneas during sleep in infants: possible relationship with sudden infant death syndrome. Science 190:677, 1975
4. Oommen PM, Roberts JL, Thach BT: Pharyngeal airway obstruction in preterm infants during mixed and obstructive apnea. J Pediatr 100:964, 1982
5. Daily WJ, Klaus M, Meyer HBP: Apnea in premature infants: monitoring, incidence, heart reate changes and effect of environmental temperature. Pediatrics 43:510, 1969
6. Buckfield PM: Neonatal at risk factors. NZ Med J 75:266, 1972
7. Smith ML, Milner AD: Bradycardia and associated respiratory changes in neonates. Arch Dis Child 56:645, 1981
8. Rigatto H, Brady JP, de La Torre Verduzco R: Chemoreceptor reflexes in preterm infants. II. The effect of gestational and postnatal age on the ventilatory response to inhaled carbondioxide. Pediatrics 55:614, 1975
9. Rigatto H, Brady JP: Periodic breathing and apnea in preterm infants. II. Hypoxia as a primary event. Pediatrics 50:219, 1972
10. Rigatto H, Brady JP, de La Torre Verduzco R: Chemoreceptor reflexes in preterm infants. I. The effect of gestational and postnatal age on the ventilatory response to inhalation of 100% and 15% oxygen. Pediatrics 55:604, 1975
11. Rigatto H: Apnea. In: Oh W(ed), The Newborn. Pediatric Clinics of North America, Vol 29. Saunders, Philadelphia, p 5, 1982
12. Martin RJ, Okken A, Rubin D: Arterial oxygen tension during active and quiet sleep in the normal neonate. J Pediat 94:271, 1979

114

13. Hanson N, Okken A: Transcutaneos oxygen tension of newborn infants in different behavioural states. Pediatr Res 14:91, 1980

14. Knill R, Bryan AC: An intercostal-phrenic inhibitory reflex in human newborn infants. J Appl Physiol 40:352, 1976

15. Boychuck RB, Seshia MMK, Rigatto H: The effect of gestational age on the effective elastance of the respiratory system. Pediatr Res 11:797, 1977

16. Bryan AC: Diaphragmatic fatique in newborns. Am Rev Resp Dis 119:143, 1979

17. Heymann MA, Rudolph AM, Silverman NH: Closure of the ductus arteriosus in premature infants by inhibition of prostaglandin synthesis. N Engl J Med 295:530, 1976

18. Fanaroff AA, Martin RJ: The respiratory system: other pulmonary problemes. In: Fanaroff AA, Martin RJ (ed), Behrman's Neonatal-perinatal Medicine: Diseases of the Fetus and Infant, 3rd ed. Mosby, St Louis, 1983

19. Perlstein H, Edward NH, Sutherland J: Apnea in premature infants and incubator air temperature changes. N Engl J Med 282:461, 1970

20. Korner AF, Kraemer HC, Haffner ME et al.: Effects of waterbed flotation on premature infants: a pilot study. Pediatrics 56:361, 1975

21. Marshall TA, Kattwinkel MD: Functional residual capacity and oxygen tension in apnea of prematurity. J Pediatr 98:479, 1981

22. Aranda JV, Sitar DS, Parson WD et al.: Pharmacokinetic aspects of theophylline in premature newborns. N Engl J Med 295:413, 1976

23. Okken A, Rubin IL, Martin RJ: Intermittent bag ventilation of preterm infants on continuous positive airway pressure: the effect on transcutaneous PO_2. J Pediatr 93:279, 1978

11. REYE'S SYNDROME – A MODERN MEDICAL MYSTERY

James P. Orlowski

INTRODUCTION

Reye's syndrome is one of man's modern medical mysteries. Despite over twenty years since it was first described and ten years of intensive study, we still have little or no idea of its pathophysiology and have succeeded in making only a minimum dent in its mortality.

HISTORICAL ASPECTS

Reye's syndrome was first described in 1963 when Ralph Douglas Kenneth Reye, the Director of The Institute of Pathology at the Royal Alexandra Hospital for

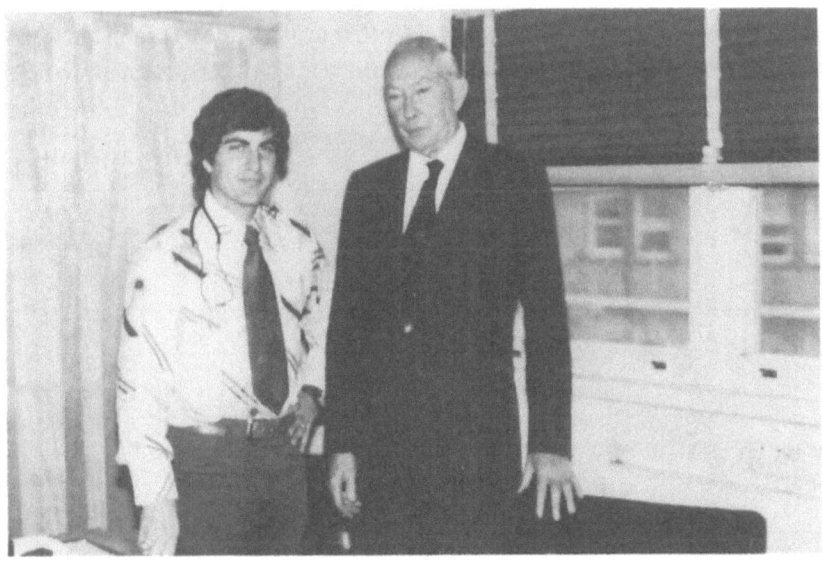

Figure 1. A photograph of Dr R.D.K. Reye (right) and the author (left). Dr Douglas Reye died on July 16, 1977, a few months after this picture was taken.

Sick Children in Sydney, Australia, described in the Lancet twenty-one children whom he had seen between 1951 and 1962 with a disease which he described as 'an encephalopathy with fatty degeneration of the viscera' (1). There have been only minor improvements in his clinical and pathologic description of this disease entity in childhood in the twenty years since his original description. In the same year of 1963 Dr G.M. Johnson and colleagues (2) described sixteen fatal cases of an encephalitis-like disease in North Carolina children, which appears to be the same syndrome.

CLINICAL PRESENTATION AND COURSE

Reye's syndrome is a life-threatening disease that develops rapidly in some children usually following an acute viral illness. It is not a common illness, with an annual incidence in the United States of less than one case per 100 000 children under the age of seventeen years.

The typical clinical course consists of a prodromal viral illness (usually Influenza A, Influenza B or varicella) which lasts for three to five days. The patient then experiences a transient period of recovery of one to three days duration, followed by the abrupt onset of protracted vomiting, which is believed to be the first sign of Reye's syndrome. Protracted vomiting is defined as emeses of more than five times in a period of eight hours. The patient then develops signs of encephalopathy with delirium alternating with stupor and it is at this time that the vomiting subsides. The patient may recover at any stage of the illness or may progress to coma with decerebration or flaccidity. Death is usually due to brainstem dysfunction and intracranial hypertension. Recovery, when it occurs, is usually complete.

Table 1. Reye's syndrome National Statistics.

Year	Cases	Deaths	% Fatal	Influenza Influenza	Incidence per 100 000 <17 yrs age
1973–74	379	157	41%	B	.58
1976–77	454	156	42%	B	.71
1977–78	237	66	29%	A (H_3N_2)	.37
1978–79	389	113	32%	A (H_1N_1)	.62
1979–80	548	114	22%	B	.88[a]
1980–81	313	89	30%	A (H_1N_1, H_3N_2)	.49
1981–82	222	73	35%	B	.35
1982–83	191	56	32%	A (H_3N_2)	.30

[a] Highest incidence occurred in 1979–80 in Ohio and Michigan with 3.5 cases/100 000 but most were stage 0 and 1 Lovejoy (stage 1 and 2 clinical staging).

If untreated the period from the start of vomiting to death is usually three to five days. Approximately 20 to 40% of Reye's syndrome cases are fatal (Table 1). The laboratory findings in Reye's syndrome are those of hepatic dysfunction. The serum transaminases are elevated consistently with the SGPT (serum glutamic pyruvate transaminase) being greater than two times normal in 99% of cases and the SGOT (serum glutamic oxaloacetic transaminase) being greater than three times normal in 95% of the cases (3). The blood ammonia level is greater than three times normal in 90% of the cases and the prothrombin time is less than 80% of normal in 79% of the cases (3). Bilirubin is elevated greater than 2 mg/dl in only 24% of cases and hypoglycemia with a blood glucose less than 40 mg/dl occurs in only 18% of cases (3). The age distribution for Reye's syndrome cases is shown in Table 2 (4).

Table 2. Age distribution.

Age in years	Percent of cases
<1	15
1–2	7
3–4	10
5–6	14
7–8	16
9–10	10
11–12	17
13–14	10
15–16	4
	100%

Cases of Reye's syndrome are divided almost equally among boys and girls. A racial breakdown indicates that white children are effected at a higher rate, although Reye's syndrome also occurs in blacks, hispanics, and other ethnic groups. Among babies under the age of one year, black infants have a higher incidence of Reye's syndrome, yet black children over the age of one year seem less susceptible to developing the disease than white children. Seizures occur in only 17% of Reye's syndrome patients older than 12 months of age, but occur in 100% of patients under the age of 10 months (5). Apneas are present in over 80% of cases of Reye's syndrome which occur in children under the age of 12 months (6). The typical case of Reye's syndrome occurs in suburban, school-age, white children under the age of 18 years during the winter or early spring months when epidemics of Influenza A, Influenza B, and chickenpox normally occur. A number of clinical staging systems for Reye's syndrome have been developed (7, 8, 9). The clinical staging system agreed on at the NIH Consensus Development Conference in 1981 is shown in Table 3 (10).

Table 3. Clinical staging of Reye's syndrome.

Stages	I	II	III	IV	V
Level of consciousness	lethargy; follows verbal commands	combative/stupor; verbalizes inappropriately	coma	coma	coma
Posture	normal	normal	decorticate	decerebrate	flaccid
Response to pain	purposeful	purposeful/non purposeful	decorticate	decerebrate	none
Pupillary reaction	brisk	sluggish	sluggish	sluggish	none
oculocephalic reflex (Doll's eyes)	normal	conjugate deviation	conjugate deviation	inconsistent or absent	none

As well as permitting comparison in clinical and scientific studies of Reye's syndrome, the clinical staging system also alerts parents and physicians to desired actions in response to the development of specific neurologic signs in children as shown in Table 4.

DIAGNOSIS

The successful management of Reye's syndrome is facilitated by early diagnosis.

Table 4.

Neurologic signs	Desired response
Vomiting	Parent awareness
Lethargy	Physician awareness
Confusion	Hospitalization
Disorientation	Hospitalization
Agitation, screaming	Intensive care
Dilated pupils	Intensive care
Hyperventilation	Intensive care
Posturing - decorticate - decerebrate	Intenstive care
Flaccid state	Intensive care

If detected and treated in its beginning stages, many Reye's syndrome patients can and do recover completely. Children who develop persistent vomiting following recovery from a viral illness and who develop listlessness, irritability, disorientation, or increasing lethargy, should receive prompt medical attention. The physician should obtain a case history and perform laboratory tests to consider the possibility of other illnesses whose symptoms mimic those of Reye's syndrome (Table 5) (11). A diagnosis of Reye's syndrome is usually made when the case history, clinical course, and laboratory findings are consistent with such a diagnosis. The laboratory tests should show evidence of an acute hepatic insult with an acute noninflammatory encephalopathy. The typically abnormal liver studies include the SGOT, SGPT, blood ammonia, and prothrombin time. There is a correlation between the admission and peak blood ammonia levels and the severity of clinical illness, with blood ammonia levels in excess of 300 μmol/L indicating more severe disease (12). There is even a better correlation with plasma lactate levels, with plasma lactate levels greater than or equal to 8 μmol/L

Table 5. Diseases which can mimic Reye's syndrome.

1) Metabolic
      urea cycle defects
      systemic carnitine deficiency
      hereditary fructose intolerance
      adipic aciduria
      diabetes and hypoglycemic disorders
      autoimmune hemolytic anemia

2) Drugs, toxins and poisonings
      salicylates
      valproic acid
      acetaminophen
      hypoglycine
      aflatoxin
      tetracycline
      methyl bromide

3) Infection
      sepsis
      pneumonia
      meningitis
      encephalitis
      hepatitis
      pancreatitis

4) SIDS

being found in severe cases and plasma lactate levels less than or equal to 4 μmol/L being consistent with mild disease (13). In occasional cases a liver biopsy may be indicated in order to confirm the diagnosis of Reye's syndrome. A liver biopsy should definitely be considered in all sporadic or atypical cases, any familial or recurrent cases, and in all infants and children under three years of age (10, 14). Although the clinical diagnosis of Reye's syndrome can be made in most patients without a liver biopsy, a liver biopsy can be performed safely after correction of the coagulation abnormalities. The liver biopsy, when properly processed and interpreted not only increases the certainty of diagnosis, but is also critically important when scientifically studying etiology or evaluating new therapeutic regimens.

TREATMENT

Although there is no known cure for Reye's syndrome, intensive supportive care in a hospital with intensive care facilities and staff experienced in treating Reye's syndrome can often reverse the course of the disease. Once a diagnosis of Reye's syndrome has been made, treatment is concentrated on the control of brain swelling and intracranial hypertension through the use of drugs and monitoring measures. Even with this aggressive therapy, some children who recover from Reye's syndrome may suffer permanent brain damage. Although treatments may vary, the prognosis for children with Reye's syndrome appears to be improving. This may be attributable in part to the fact that more diagnoses of Reye's syndrome are made before children reach advanced stages of the disease, physicians now have more experience in treating the disease, and treatment is more aggressive.

The primary management of Reye's syndrome consists first and most impotantly of a high index of suspicion of the disease. A history of a recent viral illness, especially Influenza A or B or varicella and the onset of vomiting, should alert parents and physicians to the possibility of Reye's syndrome. The next step is the establishment of a provisional diagnosis by the clinical signs of lethargy or combativeness and abnormalities in the laboratory studies of SGOT, SGPT, prothrombin time, and ammonia (15). Blood glucose, serum electrolytes, and serum osmolality should also be measured (16). The third step in the primary management of Reye's syndrome is to arrange for the transfer of the child to a fully equipped and staffed intensive care unit which is experienced in treating children with Reye's syndrome. While awaiting transfer of the child to an intensive care unit, various initial treatment steps should be instituted (16). A Foley catheter should be inserted to monitor urinary output and an intravenous infusion of $D_5^{1}/_4$ normal saline at 1.5 cc/kg/hr should be started. If neurologic signs of stage 3 Reye's syndrome or beyond (Table 3) are present or if the child is rapidly deteriorating from a neurologic standpoint then 0.25 gm/kg of Mannitol should be administered intravenously over 30 min if the serum osmolarity is less than 320 mOsm (17). If the blood sugar is less than 100 mg/dl the child should be given 0.5 to 1 gm/kg of D_{25} water intravenously. The child should be given Dexamethasone in a dose of 0.5 mg/kg intravenously and a dose of 10 mg of Vitamin K either intramuscularly or intravenously.

The management of patients following admission to an intensive care unit who are beyond stage 1 now consists of fairly aggressive therapy (16). The first step is to intubate, paralyze, and mechanically ventilate the patient. Paralysis is obtained by neuromuscular blockade with d-tubocurarine or pancuronium bromide. Mechanical ventilation is performed using tidal volumes of 10 to 15 cc/kg and rates of 12 to 20 to establish a minute ventilation compatible with a $PaCO_2$ of about 25 Torr. The FiO_2 is adjusted to provide PaO_2 values of about 100 Torr.

Intracranial pressure (ICP) monitoring is instituted as soon as possible using either intraventricular, subarachnoid, or epidural catheters, and if the ICP is less than 10 Torr then one proceeds with a lumbar puncture and cerebrospinal fluid analysis and culture. Arterial cannulation is performed for monitoring of arterial blood pressure, arterial blood gases, and pH and for the ease of blood sampling. A pulmonary artery catheterization using a Swan-Ganz catheter is performed for the monitoring of pulmonary artery wedge pressure, cardiac output and core body temperature. Moderate hypothermia is established at 30 to 31°C using surface cooling (16). Urinary output and nasal gastric fluid loss are monitored carefully. Fluid intake is restricted to 1.5 cc/kg/hr using 5% dextrose and water or 5% dextrose in 0.2% sodium chloride solution. Gastric fluid losses are replaced with 5% dextrose in $^1/_2$ normal saline. The pulmonary artery wedge pressure is maintained between 3 and 5 Torr using boluses of fluid to bring up a low pulmonary artery wedge pressure and doses of furosemide of 0.2 to 0.4 mg/kg to promote diuresis if the pulmonary artery wedge pressure exceeds 6 to 7 Torr. The plasma protein oncotic pressure is maintained above 20 Torr by using 25%

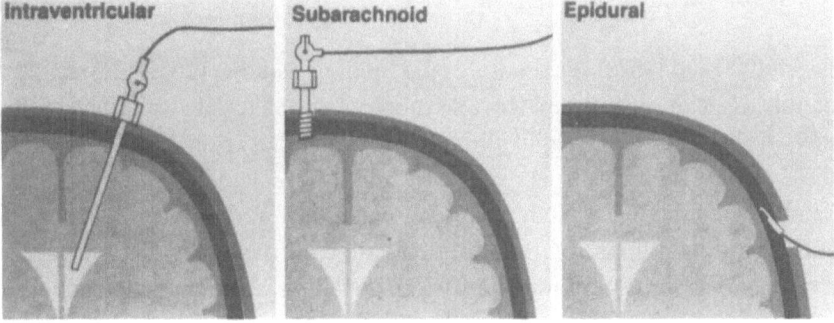

Figure 2. Depictions of intracranial pressure monitoring devices available: left: intraventricular catheter; middle: subarachnoid catheter or bolt (Richmond screw); and right: epidural catheter (Ladd monitor).

albumin infusions and the serum osmolarity is maintained between 290 and 310 mOsm. If the ICP exceeds 20 Torr, it is treated initially with manual hyperventilation for a few minutes. If the ICP remains above 20 Torr, then a does of 0.25 to 0.5 gm/kg of Mannitol (17) may be administered over 15 min and if repeated problems with elevated ICP recur then the use of barbiturates should be considered. The EKG should be continuously monitored and an EEG obtained at least once daily. The patient should be continued on Dexamethasone and Vitamin K and laboratory tests should be repeated at least once daily. It is imporant to remember that the encephalopathy of Reye's syndrome is not always associated with increased ICP (18).

Small doses of thiopental, 2 to 2.5 mg/kg, repeated as needed, once or twice per hour, are often helpful in reducing mild elevations of ICP or in preventing reaction to maneuvers known to increase ICP such as tracheal suctioning or painful stimuli, provided that systolic blood pressure is not below 80 mmHg.

Marshall et al. (19) reported good results in advanced Reye syndrome with elevated ICP when the patients were treated with a regimen incorporating the use of pentobarbital and decreased doses of Mannitol. The dose and rate of administration of the initial and subsequent doses of pentobarbital were guided by the mean cerebral perfusion pressure (50 mmHg or above) and/or blood barbiturate levels of 2.5 to 4 mg/dl. Initial dose proposed was 3 to 5 mg/kg with subsequent hourly doses of 2 to 3.5 mg/kg. Barbiturates were withheld if mean arterial pressure was less than 50 mmHg and/or blood barbiturate levels exceeded 4 mg/dl. Mannitol was only used as required by elevation of ICP above 20 mmHg which could not be controlled by the pentobarbital. We believe that this regimen provides the most rational therapy for patients with prolonged elevations of ICP.

Prognostic scoring systems have been developed which predict morbidity and mortality on the basis of ICP (16).

REYE'S SYNDROME AND SALICYLATES

Between 1980 and 1982 three separate epidemiologic studies (20, 21,22) suggested a possible association between Reye's syndrome and salicylate use. Each of these case control studies was fraught with the problems characteristic of case control studies, namely their retrospective nature and the recall ability of the parents to remember precisely what medications were administered to their children prior to and during the illness. Of the reported case control studies, only the second year of the Ohio study permitted analysis of the administration of medications on a daily basis in order to discern which drugs were administered before the onset of Reye's syndrome. Despite being the best of the reported case control studies, there are a number of very serious problems with the Ohio Department of Health Study, which make any firm conclusions about an association between salicylates and Reye's syndrome tenuous at best. The death rate in the Ohio Department of

Health Study was only 5% (22) compared to a national average of 20 to 40% (23) (Table 1) and only 19% of cases in the Ohio Department of Health Study were biopsy confirmed, which raises questions about whether many of the cases were indeed Reye's syndrome. There was also no confirmation of the medications which the parents reported having administered to their children in terms of samples of the medication or blood levels drawn on the patients. It is a well-known fact to many physicians that parents refer to acetaminophen as 'liquid aspirin'. The prevalence of fever was significantly greater in cases than in controls which may have affected the use of salicylates (24). It is also important to note that the classic biphasic cases, that is cases in which at least a one-day period between the symptoms of the antecedent illness and the onset of Reye's syndrome when no symptoms were recorded, did not use salicylates in the first three days of their illness to any significantly greater extent than their controls (24). Allegations of bias and case selection (25) have been answered by the authors of the Ohio Study (26) but are contradicted by reports from the Food and Drug Administration (27).

It is clear that not all children taking salicylates for symptoms of flu or chickenpox develop Reye's syndrome and that cases of Reye's syndrome have been identified in which no salicylates were used.

On the basis of these case control studies the Department of Health and Human Services and the Food and Drug Administration had proposed labeling precautions on all salicylate-containing drug products (24). There are a number of problems with these proposed labeling precautions, not the least of which is the impact which such labeling would have on physicians and parents. Aspirin is the standard by which all antipyretics, analgesics, and anti-inflammatory agents are compared (28). There is also the implication that acetaminophen is safe and yet experience with aspirin and acetaminophen poisonings suggest that acetaminophen may be a much more dangerous poisoning, especially because of its relative lack of symptoms in the immediate time period after ingestion when treatment is effective (29, 30). Such labeling precautions would also prevent the performance of a properly done and well-controlled study. There is also concern with the anxiety-provoking impact that such labeling precautions would have on the juvenile rheumatoid arthritis population.

Fortunately, the proposed labeling was succesfully blocked, pending the results of a well-performed study. It is interesting to note that the incidence of Reye's syndrome dramatically decreased in the 1982–1983 season (Table 1) without warning labels on aspirin ever having been instituted. The reduced number of cases probably reflects the Influenza A (H_3N_2) predominance in that year, which is less associated with Reye's syndrome than Influenza B (23). Alternatively, Reye's syndrome may be disappearing from the scene because the number of cases has steadily declined in the last 4 years despite increased physician and public awareness of the disease.

124

CONCLUSION

Reye's syndrome is a disease of childhood consisting of encephalopathy and fatty infiltration of the liver. Despite over 20 years since its original description, the etiology and pathophysiology of Reye's syndrome are still a mystery. The most important factors in the successful management of patients with Reye's syndrome are early recognition and immediate implementation of supportive therapy. In advanced or advancing cases, the therapy consists of endotracheal intubation, neuromuscular paralysis, mechanical ventilation, invasive monitoring of hemo-dynamics and intracranial pressure, and specific therapy directed at intracranial hypertension when it exists. The indiscriminate use of osmotherapy is not recommended. The preferred treatments for intracranial hypertension refractory to hyperventilation, include furosemide, thiopental, moderate hypothermia and barbiturate coma. A breakthrough in etiology and treatment of Reye's syndrome is anxiously awaited.

REFERENCES

1. Reye RDK, Morgan G, Baral J: Encephalopathy and fatty degeneration of the viscera: a disease entity in childhood. Lancet 2:749–752, 1963.
2. Johnson GM, Scurletis TD, Carroll NB: A study of sixteen fatal cases of encephalitis-like disease in North Carolina children. N C Med J 24:464–473, 1963.
3. Corey L, Rubin RJ, Bergman D et al.: Diagnostic criteria for Influenza B-associated Reye's syndrome: clinical vs. pathologic criteria. Pediatrics 60:702–714, 1977.
4. Nelson DB, Hurwitz ES, Sullivan-Bolya JZ et al.: Reye's syndrome in the United Staes in 1977–1978, a non-Influenza B virus year. J Infect Dis 140:436–439, 1979.
5. Sullivan-Bolya JZ, Nelson DB, Morens DM et al.: Reye's syndrome in children less than one year old: some epidemiologic observations. Pediatrics 65:627–629, 1980.
6. Huttenlocher PR, Trauner DA: Reye's syndrome in infancy. Pediatrics 62:84–90, 1978.
7. Huttenlocher PR: Reye's syndrome: relation of outcome to therapy. J Pediatr 80:845–850, 1972.
8. Lovejoy FH Jr, Smith AL, Bresnan MJ et al.: Clinical staging in Reye syndrome. Am J Dis Child 128:36–41,1974.
9. Aoki Y, Lombroso CT: Prognostic value of electroencephalography in Reye's syndrome. Neurology 23:333–343, 1973.
10. Consensus Conference: Diagnosis and treatment of Reye's syndrome. JAMA 246:2441–2444, 1981.
11. Crocker JFS, Bagnell PC: Reye's syndrome: a clinical review. CMA Journal 124:375–382, 1981.
12. Schubert WK, Partin JC, Partin JS: Encephalopathy and fatty liver (Reye's syndrome). Prog Liver Dis 4:489–510, 1972.
13. DeVivo DC: Reye syndrome: a metabolic response to an acute mitochondrial insult? Neurology 28:105–108, 1978.
14. Partin JC: Reye's syndrome (encephalopathy and fatty liver): diagnosis and treatment. Gastroenterology 69:511–518, 1975.
15. DeVivo DC, Keating JP, Haymond MW: Reye syndrome: results of intensive supportive care. J Pediatr 87:875–880, 1975.
16. Boutros AR, Esfandiari S, Orlowski JP et al.: Reye syndrome: a predictably curable disease. Ped Clinics NA 27:539–552, 1980.

17. Orlowski JP: Mannitol crosses the blood-brain barrier in Reye's syndrome. Cleve Clin Q 49:119–125, 1982.

18. Boutros A, Hoyt J, Menezes A et al.: Management of Reye's syndrome – a rational approach to a complex problem. Crit Care Med 5:234–238, 1977.

19. Marshall LF, Shapiro HM, Rauscher A et al.: Pentobarbital therapy for intracranial hypertension in metabolic coma - Reye's syndrome. Crit Care Med 6:1–5, 1978.

20. Starko KM, Ray CG, Dominguez LB et al.: Reye's syndrome and salicylate use. Pediatrics 66:859–864, 1980.

21. Waldman RJ, Hall WN, McGee H et al.: Aspirin as a risk factor in Reye's syndrome. JAMA 247:3089–3099, 1982.

22. Halpin TJ, Holtzhauer FJ, Campbell RJ et al.: Reye's syndrome and medication use. JAMA 248:687–691, 1982.

23. Hurwitz ES, Nelson DB, Davis C et al.: National surveillance for Reye syndrome: a five-year review. Pediatrics 70:895–900, 1982.

24. Department of Health and Human Services: labeling for salicylate-containing drug products; advance notice of proposed rulemaking. Fed Reg 47:57885–57901, 1982.

25. Orlowski JP: Aspirin and Reye's syndrome (letter to editor). JAMA 249:3177, 1983.

26. Halpin TJ, Holtzhauer FJ, Campbell RJ et al.: Aspirin and Reye's syndrome (reply). JAMA 249:3177, 1983.

27. Department of Health and Human Services: Food and Drug Administration. Fed Reg 47:57892, 1982.

28. Lovejoy FH Jr: Aspirin and acetaminophen: a comparative view of their antipyretic and analgesic activity. Pediatrics 62:904–909, 1978.

29. American Academy of Pediatrics Committee on Drugs: Commentary on acetaminophen. Pediatrics 61:108–112, 1978.

30. Rumack BH: Aspirin versus acetaminophen: a comparative view. Pediatrics 62:943–946, 1978.

12. CONTINUOUS MONITORING OF PO_2 AND PCO_2

Hans T. Versmold

INTRODUCTION

The invention of simple electrochemical sensors for measuring partial pressures of oxygen (1) and of carbon dioxide (2, 3) has opened a new field in medicine, and particularly in intensive care medicine. Later, continuous rather than intermittent monitoring of blood gases has added important information to respiratory physiology and to clinical care, particularly to neonatal intensive care. The major practical impacts of continuous blood gas monitoring are:

1. We can detect rapid changes in both oxygenation (PaO_2) and ventilation ($PaCO_2$), allowing immediate onset of diagnostic and therapeutical approaches.
2. We have learned, how great a variability there is in the blood gases of healthy and sick infants, and how little a single value of PO_2 or PCO_2 taken at a random point in time really tells us about an infant's long-term state of oxygenation and/ or ventilation. We may, therefore, miss or erroneously assume hypoxemia or hyperoxemia, hypokapnia or hyperkapnia. A wrong 'treatment' will then be done on the basis of the misleading intermittent blood gas determination.

    The unsettled issue of retinopathy of prematurity, for example, awaits complete reevaluation using the new techniques of long-term continuous monitoring of PO_2 and PCO_2.
3. Noninvasive monitoring is an important part of the principle of 'minimal handling' which should reduce the risk of intracranial hemorrhage in the very low birth weight infant.

    The focus of this contribution is on noninvasive continuous blood gas monitoring, but it includes a brief evaluation of invasive methods to monitor oxygenation and ventilation.

MONITORING OF PO_2

It must be kept in mind that arterial PO_2 (PaO_2) is only one of the variables determining arterial oxygen content, and thus – besides cardiac output – determining systemic oxygen transport. Other important factors include the oxygen-carrying capacity of blood, i.e. hemoglobin concentration, and the oxygen affinity of blood (P50 value), depending mainly on pH, PCO_2, red cell 2,3-DPG levels, and the presence of fetal or adult hemoglobin (4). Therefore, the PaO_2 necessary to assure a hemoglobin oxygen saturation of 90% ('P90') increases with gestational age. Table 1 shows such 'P90' values. Monitoring PaO_2 alone, without considering these factors, is therefore inadequate (5).

In the neonate, capillary PO_2 arteriolar PO_2 do not reliably reflect PaO_2 (6, 7); even after heating or application of vasodilating drugs to the skin there is an unpredictable amount of venous admixture to the sample making capillary PO_2 monitoring an obsolete method for monitoring the arterial oxygenation state. Tissue oxygen supply may be better reflected by mixed venous PO_2, or to some extent by skin surface PO_2.

Table 1. PO_2 needed for 90% oxygen saturation.[a]

Gestational age	P90[a]
26 wks	47 Torr
32 wks	50 Torr
40 wks	52 Torr
40+4 wks	54 Torr
40+8 wks	59 Torr

[a] At pH 7.4 and 37°C

Intermittent PO_2 monitoring in arterial blood samples

Arterial blood samples drawn through an umbilical aortic catheter with the tip below the level of the ductus arteriosus will provide information about the PaO_2 in the postductal part of the circulation. This PaO_2 may be lower than that reaching the head and eyes if there is right to left shunting through the ductus. From the difference between preductal and postductal PaO_2 the extent of ductal right to left shunting can be estimated (8).

Blood sampling through a (right) radial or temporal artery stick will provide the more relevant information on the preductal PO_2. Sampling, however, has to be finished within 10–15 sec, i.e. within one circulation time, because pain and crying increase intrathoracic pressure, increase atrial (and ductal) shunting, thereby leading to a fall in PaO_2 both in the pre- and postductal circulation.

Blood pressure spikes associated with the painful arterial puncture may be directly transmitted to the cerebral circulation in case of a disturbed autoregulation of cerebral blood flow (9), e.g. after asphyxia or apnea.

Continuous monitoring of PO₂

Reliable oxygen electrodes are now manufactured both for continuous intravascular PaO_2 monitoring and for continuous monitoring of PO_2 noninvasively on the skin surface.

Intravascular PO₂ monitoring. A minuaturized PO_2 electrode for intravascular PO_2 monitoring imbedded in the tip of an umbilical artery catheter (10) is now available for clinical routine use. In our hands there was excellent agreement between the catheter tip PO_2 and PaO_2 values measured in blood samples drawn through the catheter lumen (11) (Figure 1). The catheter tip electrode is stable in situ so that recalibration is necessary only once a day (12). As expected, this direct method of PaO_2 monitoring is unaffected by the infants clinical condition, allowing reliable PaO_2 registration also in shock. The catheters have a side hole in contrast to the end hole of conventional catheters, but both the 4F and 5F catheter allow accurate undamped monitoring of blood pressure (12). In our experience, though, the 4F catheter had a tendency of being obstructed earlier.

Not recommended for use in neonates is another system designed for intravascular PO_2 monitoring in adults (Hoffmann-La Roche, Basel). This PO_2 electrode can be passed through a 5F catheter and PO_2 monitoring is possible. However the anode of the electrode is 5 cm distal to its tip so that the electrode has to look out of the catheter that far. This implies that in the neonate either the catheter tip or the electrode tip must be positioned at a dangerous level of the aorta.

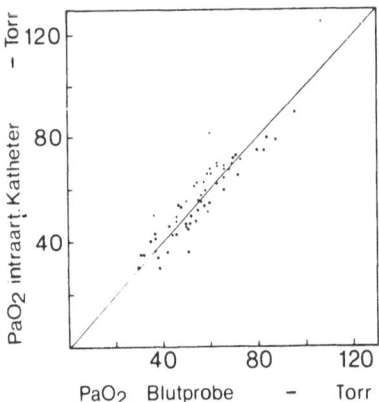

Figure 1. Relation between arterial PO₂ measured by a catheter tip electrode (Searle, High Wycombe, UK) in the abdominal aorta and PaO₂ in blood sampled through the catheter (adapted from Ref. 11).

Skin surface PO$_2$ monitoring

Skin surface PO$_2$ (tcPO$_2$) in newborn infants closely reflects PaO$_2$, when the skin is heated to 44°C for vasodilatation (13, 14). This agreement between tcPO$_2$ and PaO$_2$ results from the fortunate fact that various factors determining the skin surface PO$_2$ under the heated electrode are balancing each other: heating causes an increase of capillary PO$_2$ by vasodilatation and arterialization of capillary blood, by the anaerobic heating coefficient, and by the right shift of the hemoglobin oxygen equilibrium curve. On the other hand, there is a fall in PO$_2$ as it diffuses to the skin surface, by the oxygen consumption of the epidermis, and by the electrode itself. By chance, and so only in newborn and young infants, tcPO$_2$ is virtually identical with PaO$_2$.

When we applied four different tcPO$_2$ electrodes (Huch prototype, Draeger-Hellige, Radiometer, Roche; all at 44° C) simultaneously to the skin of newborn infants, all tcPO$_2$ values agreed equally well with PaO$_2$ ($r = 0.98$). Also, their response times in situ to a step change in the concentration of inspired oxygen (FiO$_2$) were not different among the microcathode and macrocathode electrodes, despite large differences in their in vitro response times (15). tcPO$_2$ follows PaO$_2$ with a delay of 15–30 sec which is mainly due to damping by the skin and not by the electrode (15). This implies that swings in tcPO$_2$, as they occur e.g. during handling (16), are only damped reflections of larger swings in PaO$_2$.

Problems with tcPO$_2$ monitoring and what they can tell us. As expected, during severely impaired peripheral perfusion tcPO$_2$ does no longer reflect PaO$_2$ (17). Blood pressure (BP), among the variables analyzed (BP, blood volume, hematocrit, viscosity, pH musculocutaneous blood flow of a leg (Figures 2 and 3)), predicted best whether tcPO$_2$ (44° C) agreed with PaO$_2$ or not. If blood pressure deviates below the 95% confidence limits of normal (18), too low a tcPO$_2$ is to be expected: below 35 mmHg of systolic blood pressure, the mean ratio of tcPO$_2$/PaO$_2$ was 0.6 (Figure 2A). A tcPO$_2$ below PaO$_2$ is therefore an important information. It strongly suggests a severely impaired cardiocirculatory state with impaired tissue oxygen supply. In such infants PaO$_2$ must be monitored invasively (19).

tcPO$_2$ monitoring may cause skin lesions, mainly by the adhesive ring which has to be changed every 3–4 hr, and by the heat if there is poor peripheral perfusion. These problems are more frequent in the very low birth weight infant. Even this problem may turn into an information: the intensity of such red spots can be used as a clinical sign of alarm. Even moderate changes in microcirculation, e.g. with the onset of sepsis, go along with more pronounced and prolonged heat marks on the skin.

tcPO$_2$ and apnea. Among the clinical states at which there is a discrepancy between tcPO$_2$ and PaO$_2$, the recovery phase after an apneic attack is an example

131

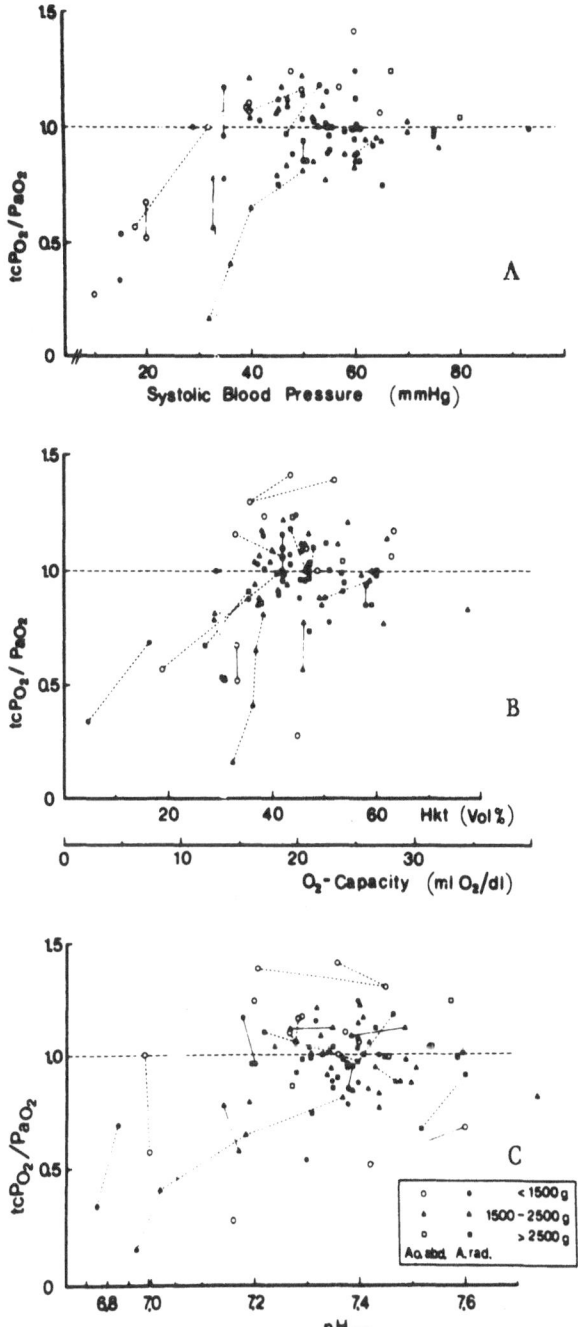

Figure 2. Influence of systolic blood pressure, O_2 capacity (hematocrit), arterial pH on the ratio of tcPO$_2$ (44°C)/PaO$_2$ in sick neonates (adapted from Ref. 17).

132

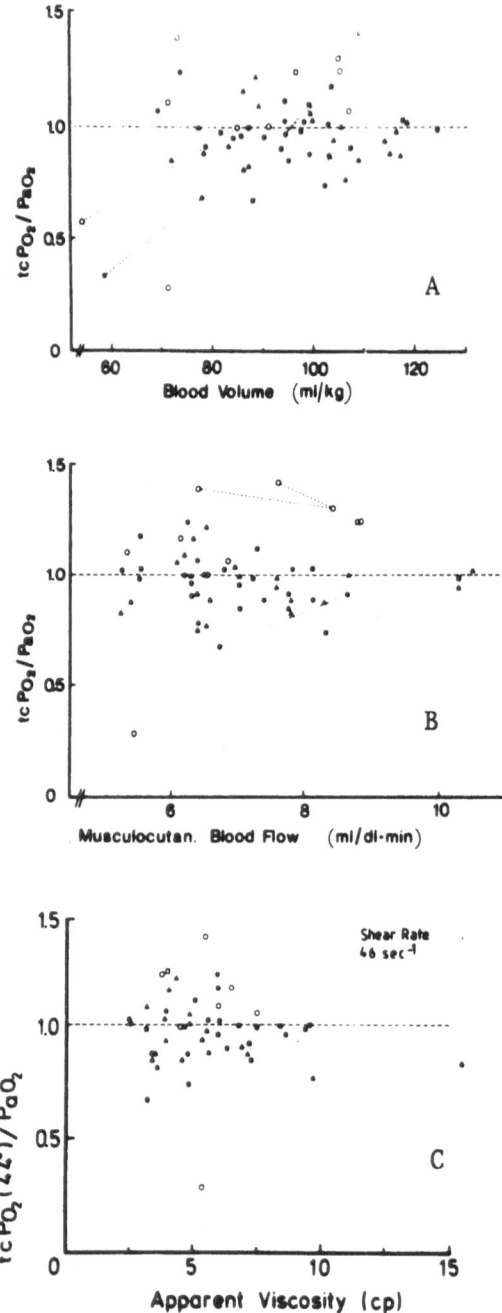

Figure 3. Influence of blood volume, musculocutaneous blood flow of a leg, and apparent viscosity on the ratio of tcPO$_2$ (44° C)/PaO$_2$ in sick neonates (adapted from Ref. 17).

of particular importance. After a severe apneic attack PaO_2 may be low for several reasons (right to left shunting, decreased alveolar ventilation, and others) requiring increased FiO_2. Dosage of oxygen is usually controlled by $tcPO_2$ in such situations. However a pronounced vasoconstriction after an apneic attack often persists for 10–15 min after restitution of regular breathing and may lead to significant underestimation of PaO_2 by $tcPO_2$, resulting in the use of too high a FiO_2 and critically high PaO_2 values. An example is given in Figure 4.

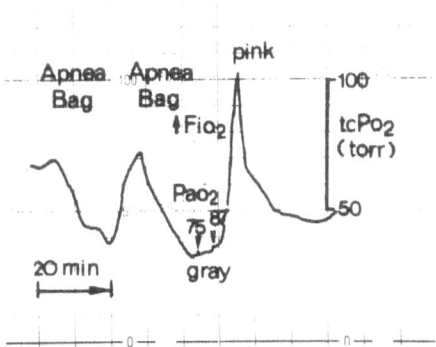

Figure 4. Low $tcPO_2$ despite high PaO_2 after a severe apneic attack, while the infant looks gray and pale for 15 min. In an attempt to normalize $tcPO_2$, FiO_2 was increased leading to arterial hyperoxemia.

Alarm limits of PaO_2 ($tcPO_2$). Normal values of PaO_2 in term (20, 36) and preterm (21) neonates are given in Table 2. PaO_2 ($tcPO_2$) should be kept above 50 Torr, i.e. in a range to assure a 90% oxygen saturation of hemoglobin (Table 1). In the very low birth weight infant, at high levels of fetal hemoglobin, 45 Torr may assure a suffucient arterial oxygen content, provided hematocrit and pH are normal. We set the upper limits of PaO_2 to 70 Torr, not because of a risk of retinopathy, but because a higher PaO_2 is unnecessary, is obtained by too high a

Table 2. Arterial blood gas tensions in healthy neonates.[a]

	24 hr	36 hr	7 d
	M ± SD (range)	M ± SD (range)	M ± SD (range)
PaO_2 (Torr)			
Term[b]	72 ± 7 (62–91)	74 ± 8 (62–91)	74 ± 7 (62–91)
Preterm	67 ± 15	72 ± 21	80 ± 12
$PaCO_2$ (Torr)			
Term	35 ± 3 (30–41)	33 ± 3 (26–43)	37 ± 3 (30–42)
Preterm	27 ± 8	31 ± 7	36 ± 4

[a] Mean (M) and standard deviation (SD). Data from Ref. 20 (term infants) and Ref. 21 (preterm infants).
[b] $tcPO_2$ at 6–12 hr (36): mean of infants' highest $tcPO_2$ 89 ± 11 Torr, lowest $tcPO_2$ 78 ± 12 Torr.

FiO$_2$, with an increasing, risk of bronchopulmonary dysplasia. PaO$_2$ values above 90 Torr should be strictly avoided because of the risk of retinopathy.

The consideration of the above mentioned limitations and advantages of tcPO$_2$ monitoring should lead to the safer use of this method, which probably has been the most important contribution improving the quality of neonatal care during the last decade.

MONITORING OF PCO$_2$

Monitoring of PaCO$_2$ is of similar importance as monitoring of PaO$_2$. Mechanical ventilation of newborn infants today aims at keeping PaCO$_2$ within more narrow normal limits, mainly because PCO$_2$ controls cerebral and retinal blood flow. Various problems associated with hyperkapnia and hypokapnia are listed in Table 3.

Table 3. Why PaCO$_2$ monitoring?

Problems associated with hyperkapnia
– Cerebral congestion, risk of bleeding
– Retinal vasodilatation, risk of retinopathy
– Pulmonary vascular resistance increases
– Renal blood flow decreased
– Dyspnea
– Acidemia, electrolyte imbalance

Problems associated with hypokapnia
– Cerebral blood flow reduced
– Hypotension
– Apnea
– Alkalemia, electrolyte imbalance
– Acutely: low P50

Intermittent PCO$_2$ monitoring

Capillary PCO$_2$ values are about 5 Torr higher on the first day, but correlate closely to arterial values (unlike PO$_2$), provided peripheral blood flow is not severely disturbed and the skin is warmed prior to sampling. Capillary PCO$_2$ is therefore acceptable to monitor alveolar ventilation, and to verify continuous skin surface PCO$_2$ monitoring. The main disadvantage is the intermittent information requiring frequent painful punctures with the potential risks already discussed.

Continuous PCO$_2$ monitoring

Sensors for *intravascular* continuous PCO$_2$ monitoring (mass spectroscopy, electrochemical sensors) are as yet not ready for routine clinical application. *Endexspiratory PCO$_2$*, useful in the adult and healthy newborn, does not reflect PaCO$_2$ in the newborn with major respiratory problems. *Skin surface PCO$_2$* monitoring is just becoming a clinical tool. Both with mass spectrometry and infrared analysis preliminary results were obtained. However, PCO$_2$ electrodes appear to be the simplest technique for clinical routine use (22, 25).

Skin surface PCO$_2$ monitoring. By a miniaturized heated PCO$_2$ electrode on the skin PaCO$_2$ can be estimated continuously (26, 27). This PCO$_2$ electrode (23), like any PCO$_2$ electrode, sonsists of a micro glass pH electrode dipped into a bicarbonate solution and covered with a Teflon membrane permeable to CO$_2$. A change in ambient PCO$_2$ alters the pH beneath the electrode which is measured. The electrodes are calibrated in 5% and 10% CO$_2$ gas (23).

We found a close linear correlation between tcPCO$_2$ and PaCO$_2$, using the same electrode temperature (44°C) as for tcPO$_2$ monitoring. Also at 41°C, 42°C and 43°C was tcPCO$_2$ closely related to PaCO$_2$ (Table 4) (24, 26).

tcPCO$_2$ is higher than PaCO$_2$ because the anaerobic heating coefficient and the local CO$_2$ production by the skin add up resulting in a PCO$_2$ on the skin surface about 1.5 times that in arterial blood (23). An adjustment can be applied to the calibration of tcPO$_2$ electrodes so that the displayed PCO$_2$ corresponds to the actual arterial values (28). For clinical practice, we set the displayed PCO$_2$ in 5% CO$_2$ to 20 Torr, in 10% CO$_2$ to 50 Torr (at any electrode temperature from 41–44°C) accepting a small error.

The close correlations between tcPO$_2$ and PaCO$_2$ (41–44°C) were unaffected by systolic BP down to below 25 mmHg (Figure 5) (28). As compared to PO$_2$, skin surface PCO$_2$ is obviously less dependent on skin perfusion (Figure 6). However, experience in infants with cardiogenic shock (29), and during severe metabolic acidosis (30), like in our infants with systolic blood pressure below 15 mmHg, showed elevated tcPO$_2$ values (44°C) up to 3 times above PaCO$_2$. On the other

Table 4. Linear regression equations of the relation between skin surface PCO$_2$ (y; Torr) and arterial PCO$_2$ (x; Torr).

Temperature	Equation[a]	N	r	s_{xy} [b]
41°C	y = 1.24× + 9.00	59	0.87	3.57
43°C	y = 1.26× + 9.86	88	0.94	3.20
44°C	y = 1.30× + 7.20	76	0.94	3.02

[a] Data at systolic blood pressure below 15 mmHg omitted
[b] Standard error of estimate (Torr) for the prediction of PaCO$_2$ from tcPO$_2$.

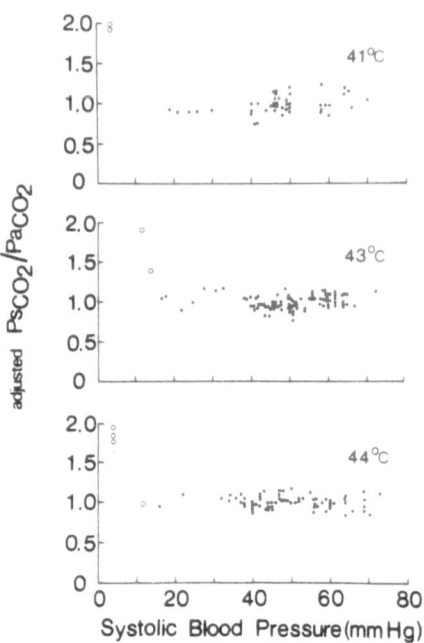

Figure 5. Influence of systolic blood pressure on the ratio of adjusted $tcPO_2/PaCO_2$ at various electrode temperatures. Note that $tcPO_2$ deviates from $PaCO_2$ at systolic blood pressures below 20 mmHg (0) (compare with $tcPO_2$, Figure 2A) (adapted from Ref. 28).

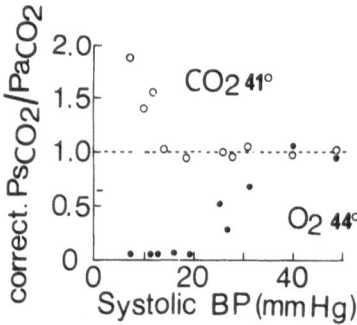

Figure 6. Ratio of tc/arterial PO_2 (0) and PCO_2 (0) during recovery from severe shock. $tcPCO_2$ agrees with $PaCO_2$ already at lower blood pressures.

hand, $tcPCO_2$ (41–44° C) correlated with $PaCO_2$ in hypothermic adults (core temperature 28–32°C) with a normal cardiac output during cardiac surgery (31). At an electrode temperature of 37° C the relation of $tcPCO_2/PaCO_2$ is more sensitive to circulatory changes (32).

The response time of various $tcPCO_2$ electrodes (Radiometer, Roche, Novametrix) is in the order of 1 min (90% response in vitro), and thus sufficient to pick up even rapid changes in $PaCO_2$ (which changes less rapidly than PaO_2). $tcPCO_2$ reacts promptly to crying, apnea, or sustained alterations of alveolar ventilation, but does not fluctuate with periodic breathing. The in situ response time increases, when a lower electrode temperature is used, At 37° C tcPCO$_2$ reacts quite slowly.

At 41°C we did not see skin burns, and the response time was still quite acceptable. In premature infants we therefore use the electrode at 41° C and recalibrate it at longer intervals (6 hr), i.e. with every second calibration of the tcPO$_2$ electrode. This low temperature needed for tcPCO$_2$ monitoring, and also the stability of the electrodes (drift less than 2 Torr/6 hr) make them suitable instruments for long-term continuous monitoring.

Alarm limits of PCO$_2$. Normal values of PaCO$_2$ in neonates (20, 21) are given in Table 2. In the preterm infant, because of the risk of intracranial hemorrhage and retinopathy, a PaCO$_2$ of 45–50 Torr is now considered and indication for mechanical ventilation. In the infant on a respirator we aim at a PaCO$_2$ of 35 Torr, with the alarm limits at 30–45 Torr. PCO$_2$ values above 45 Torr are accepted only in the older infant being weaned from the respirator.

Continuous monitoring of PCO$_2$ is of particular clinical interest. For example, it reduces the phase of trial-and-error during the initial setting of respirator, helps in the immediate evaluation of effects, e.g. of high frequency ventilation, is an early, sensitive indicator of respiratory muscle fatique during weaning, and proved extremely helpful in controlling the extent of hypokapnia (20–25 Torr), induced to reduce pulmonary vascular resistance in the persistent fetal circulation syndrome.

THE FUTURE OF MONITORING PO$_2$ AND PCO$_2$

The development of probes able to measure several gases on the skin may be the way to go in the future. Combined PO$_2$+PCO$_2$ electrodes have already been used successfully (33, 34, 35) in newborn infants, with the major advantage that only one instead of two adhesive rings has to be torn off the fragile skin for recalibration of the electrode. Theoretically, mass spectrometry should become the technique of choice, as it allows quasisimultaneous measuring of as many gases as one wishes to measure, making the skin an exciting playground for many more than only neonatologists.

CONCLUSION

Continuous monitoring of PaO$_2$ and PaCO$_2$ have reduced the short-term hazards of neonatal intensive care. They may, in the future, reduce long-term hazards like bronchopulmonary dysplasia and retinopathy of prematurity.

138

ACKNOWLEDGEMENT

The cooperation in the studies on which this report is based, by Prof. K. Riegel, Prof. O. Linderkamp, Prof. J.W. Severinghaus, Dr Ingrid Brünstler, Dr Angelika Enders and Dr M. Holzmann is gratefully acknowledged, as well as the continuous engaged help by the nurses of the Neonatal Intensive Care Nurseries in the Department of Pediatrics and the Klinikum Grosshadern of the University of Munich.

These studies were supported in part by Grant Ve 32/3 of the Deutsche Forschungsgemeinschaft.

REFERENCES

1. Clark LC Jr: Monitor and control of blood and tissue oxygen tensions. Trans Am Soc Artif Intern Organs 2:41, 1956
2. Stow RW, Bear RF, Randall BF: Arch Phys Med Rehabil 38:646, 1957
3. Severinghaus JW, Bradley AF: Electrodes for blood PO_2 and PCO_2 determination. J Appl Physiol 13:515, 1958
4. Riegel KP, Versmold HT: Respiratory gas transport characteristics of blood and hemoglobin. In: Stawe U (ed), Perinatal Physiology, 2nd ed. Plenum Med Book Co, New York, London p 241, 1978
5. Duc G: Assessment of hypoxia in the newborn. Suggestions for a practical approach. Pediatrics 48:469, 1971
6. Koch G, Wendel H: Comparison of pH, carbon dioxide tension, standard bicarbonate and oxygen tension in capillary blood during the neonatal period. Acta Paed Scand 56:10, 1967
7. Duc G, Curasamy N: Digital arteriolar oxygen tension as a guide to oxygen therapy of the newborn. Biol Neonate 24:134, 1974
8. Gersony WM, Duc GV, Dell RB, Sinclair JC: Oxygen method for calculation of the right to left shunt. New application in presence of right to left shunt through the ductus arteriosus . Cardiovasc Res 6:423, 1972
9. Lou HC, Lassen NA, Frits-Hansen B: Is arterial hypertension crucial for the development of intraventricular hemorrhage in the neonate? Lancet i:1215, 1979
10. Conway M, Durbin GM, Ingram D, Mc Intosh N, Parker D, Reynolds EOR, Soutter LP: Continuous monitoring of arterial oxygen tension using a catheter-tip polarographic electrode in infants. Pediatrics 57:244, 1976
11. Enders A, Linderkamp O, Riegel K, Sebening W, Versmold H: Kontinuierliche intraarterielle PO_2-Überwachung in der Neugeborenen-Intensivpflege. In: von Loewenich V (ed), Pädiatrische Intensivpflege. Enke, Stuttgart (in press)
12. Wilkinson AR, Phibbs RH, Gregory GA: Improved accuracy of continuous measurements of arterial oxygen tension in sick newborn infants. Criteria for reading and recalibrating the electrode. Arch Dis Childh 54:307, 1979
13. Huch R, Lübbers DW, Huch A: Quantitative continuous measurement of partial oxygen pressure on the skin of adults and newborn babies. Pflügers Arch 337:185, 1972
14. Eberhard P, Hammacher K, Mindt W: Perkutane Messung des Sauerstoffpartialdruckes. Proc Medizin-Technik, Stuttgart, p 26, 1972
15. Versmold HT, Linderkamp O, Stuffer KH, Holzmann M, Riegel KP: In vivo vs in vitro response time of $tcPO_2$ electrodes. A comparison of four devices in newborn. Acta Anaesth Scand Suppl. 168:40, 1978

16. Long J, Philip A, Lucey J: Excessive handling as a cause of hypoxemia. Pediatrics 65:203, 1980
17. Versmold HT, Linderkamp O, Holzmann M, Strohhacker I, Riegel KP: Transcutaneous PO_2 monitoring in sick infants. Where are the limits? Influence of blood pressure, blood volume, blood flow, viscosity and acid–base state. Birth Defects, Original Article Series (The National Foundation) XV (4):285, 1979
18. Versmold HT, Kitterman, JA, Phibbs RH, Gregory GA, Tooley WH: Aortic blood pressure durig the first 12 hours of life in infants with birth weight 610 to 4220 grams. Pediatrics 67:611, 1981
19. Riegel KP, Versmold HT: Intraarterial vs transcutaneous PO_2 monitoring in newborn infants. Biotelemetry 6:32, 1979
20. Koch G, Wendel H: Adjustment of arterial blood gases and acid–base balance in the normal newborn infant during the first week of life. Biol Neonate 12:136, 1968
21. Orzalesi MM, Mendicini M, Bucci G, Scalamandre A, Savignioni PG: Arterial oxygen studies in premature newborns with and without mild respiratory disorders. Arch Dis Childh 174, 1967
22. John RJ, Lindsay WJ, Shepard RH: A system for monitoring alveolar ventilation. Biomed Sci Instrumentation 5:119, 1969
23. Severinghaus JW, Stafford M, Bradley AF: tcPO$_2$ electrode design, calibration and temperature gradient problems. Acta Anaesth Scand Suppl 68:118, 1978
24. Huch A, Seiler D, Meinzer K, Huch R, Galster H, Lübbers DW: Transcutaneous PCO_2 measurement with a miniaturized electrode. Lancet i:118, 1979
25. Eberhard P, Schäfer R: A sensor for noninvasive monitoring of carbon dioxide. Br J Clin Equip, p 224, Nov 1980
26. Versmold HT, Severinghaus JW, Müller C, Paikert I, Riegel KP: Transcutaneous monitoring of PCO_2 in newborn infants. Pediatr Res 13:73, 1979
27. Hansen TN, Tooley WH: Skin surface carbon dioxide tension in sick infants. Pediatrics 64:942, 1979
28. Brünstler I, Enders A, Versmold HT: Skin surface PCO_2 monitoring in newborn infants in shock: effect of hypotension and electrode temperature. J Pediatr 100:454, 1982
29. Schöber JG, Stübing K: Arterial and transcutaneous PCO_2 monitoring in carciogenic shock. In: Huch R, Huch A (eds), Continuous Transcutaneous Blood Gas Monitoring. Marcel Dekker, London, New York, 1983
30. Cohen, J: Transcutaneous carbon dioxide tension in acidotic infants. In: Huch R, Huch A (eds), Continuous Transcutaneous Blood Gas Monitoring. Marcel Dekker London, New York, 1983
31. Vogel H, Madler C, Franke N, Schmucker P, Kreuzer E, Peter K, Versmold HT: Effect of hypothermia and extracorporeal circulation on transcutaneous PCO_2 readings during cardiac surgery. In: Huch R, Huch A (eds), Continuous Transcutaneous Blood Gas Monitoring. Marcel Dekker, London, New York, p 771, 1983
32. Tremper KK, Mentelos RA, Shoemaker WC: Effect of hypercarbia and shock on transcutaneous carbon dioxide at different electrode temperatures. Crit Care Med 8:608, 1980
33. Whitehead M, Halsall D, Pollitzer M, Delpy DT, Parker D, Reynolds EOR: Transcutaneous estimation of arterial PO_2 and PCO_2 in newborn infants with a single electrochemical sensor. Lancet i:1111, 1980
34. Severinghaus JW: Combined PO_2 and PCO_2 transcutaneous electrode with electrochemical HCO_3 stabilization. J Appl Physiol 51:1027, 1981
35. Huch R, Krähenmann F, Bucher HU, Huch A: First experiences with a combined PO_2-PCO_2 electrode. Proc 8th Eur Cong Perinatal Medicine, 1983
36. Huch R, Huch A, Rooth G: An Atlas of Cardiorespirograms in Newborn Infants. Wolfe Med Publ Ltd, p 217, 1983

13. GAS EXCHANGE DURING COVENTIONAL AND HIGH-FREQUENCY VENTILATION

Peter D. Wagner

Peter D. Wagner

INTRODUCTION

This chapter will highlight some important issues concerning pulmonary gas exchange during both conventional and high-frequency oscillatory ventilation. The data upon which the text is based come from the literature as well as from the author's own laboratory. In a presentation of this length, a full treatment of gas exhange is clearly infeasible, and thus only selected topics are discussed. These have been chosen because of their clinical importance. In some cases, these topics represent concepts that are well established in the physiological literature, but not generally applied in the clinical care of the patient. In others, the ideas are more recent, of great interest, but not yet completely resolved (especially the issues concerning gas exchange during high-frequency ventilation). They are presented to stimulate thought and discussion of possible approaches to solving these problems. The ideas presented in these cases are clearly speculative, but may suggest possible clarifying studies. Table 1 lists the issues that will be discussed.

Table 1. Topics covered in this chapter.

Gas exchange during conventional ventilation
1. Quantification of gas exchange abnormality by PaO_2
2. Importance of knowing mixed venous PO_2 in gas exchange analysis
3. Effect of cardiac output on PaO_2
4. FiO_2 and quantification of gas exchange abnormality

Gas exchange during high-frequency oscillatory ventilation
1. Efficacy in the presence of intrapulmonary shunting
2. Efficacy in the presence of ventilation/perfusion inequality
3. Mucociliary clearance and gas exchange

GAS EXCHANGE DURING CONVENTIONAL VENTILATION

Quantification of gas exchange by PaO$_2$

Arterial PO$_2$ is routinely used to assess the state of health of the lungs and it is generally true that under a given set of conditions, the higher the PaO$_2$, the better the lungs. However, the key to this conclusion is the caveat concerning the given set of conditions. What is crucial is to understand how PaO$_2$ is determined by many factors. These factors fall into two groups: 1) those related to the health of the lung per se (degree of shunting, ventilation/perfusion $\dot{V}_A/\dot{Q}$) mismatch and alveolar-endcapillary diffusion disequilibrium), and 2) those related to extra-pulmonary factors such as FiO$_2$, total alveolar ventilation, cardiac output, O$_2$ uptake, and less important influences such as temperature, acid-base status, hemoglobin concentration, and the shape and position of the O$_2$Hb dissociation curve. These multiple factors interact in a complicated, yet logical way that is amenable to systematic quantitative analysis (1). How this can be done was illustrated in the previous symposium in this series (2). Consequently, in analyzing PaO$_2$ as an index of the gas exchange status of the lungs per se, one must have knowledge of the extrapulmonary influences on PaO$_2$. This poses a very difficult problem in clinical practice because a large body of information, some that can be obtained *reliably* only by invasive means, must be obtained for a rigorous analysis, and in addition, one must have a feel for how much a change in any such factor will affect PaO$_2$. To the extent that both these data and analytical techniques are not pursued, one may make quite erroneous conclusions regarding the health of the lungs.

Generally, PaO$_2$ can be used to quantify the gas exchange abnormality by three traditional approaches, and it is the purpose of this section to indicate which of these is least affected by the confounding extrapulmonary influences referred to above. The first is by PaO$_2$ itself. This is the most direct, but least insightful method because it is influenced so much by changes in extrapulmonary factors. This has been known for some time. For example, Pontoppidan (3) shows how, in the presence of a constant intrapulmonary shunt, PaO$_2$ (while breathing pure O$_2$), can vary up to hundreds of Torr, depending on the cardiac output. Clearly, any inference from PaO$_2$ failing to quantitatively allow for such changes will be potentially grossly erroneous, leading to false conclusions regarding resolution of lung disease, and hence to incorrect therapeutic decisions. Equally important effects of changes in O$_2$ uptake ($\dot{V}$ O$_2$) ventilation and FiO$_2$ on PaO$_2$ are demonstrable (2).

The second approach is to use the alveolar–arterial PO$_2$ difference (A–a DO$_2$). While this variable has less dependence on total alveolar ventilation than does PaO$_2$ itself, changes in FiO$_2$ and cardiac output will significantly alter the A–a DO$_2$ even while the degree of intrapulmonary abnormality remains constant.

It turns out that of the three, the third standard approach, that of calculating venous admixture, is least affected by extrapulmonary influences. Venous admixture is easily calculated from the shunt equation knowing O_2 content in three locations: 1) arterial blood (CaO_2), 2) mixed venous blood ($C\bar{v}O_2$), and 3) endcapillary blood ($Cc'O_2$). CaO_2 is directly measured from an arterial sample (or computed from the measured PaO_2); $C\bar{v}O_2$ is derived similarly, or if mixed venous blood is not available, it is estimated by mass conservation from measured values of $\dot{V}O_2$ and cardiac output. If these variables have not been measured, $C\bar{v}O_2$ must be assumed. The consequences of this assumption will be discussed below in the next section. $Cc'O_2$ is calculated from alveolar PO_2, which is turn is computed from the alveolar gas equation (4) knowing arterial PCO_2.

Even while PaO_2 and the A–a DO_2 will vary with, say, FiO_2 or cardiac output, venous admixture will *not* if the real mixed venous PO_2 is known and if the intrapulmonary abnormality is one of shunting ($\dot{V}_A/\dot{Q}$ of zero) (2). This is a great advantage in differentiating shunting from extrapulmonary causes of hypoxemia. However, even with venous admixture, there will be dependence on FiO_2 and cardiac output, $\dot{V}O_2$ and total ventilation if the intrapulmonary abnormality is one of $\dot{V}_A/\dot{Q}$ mismatch. Thus, West (1) showed how in the face of a constant degree of $\dot{V}_A/\dot{Q}$ mismatching, venous admixture increases as cardiac output increases, and vice versa. This problem is very difficult to overcome in practice. About the best that can be done is to attempt to make venous admixture measurements under as nearly as possible the same conditions if sequential samples are to be compared. The most relevant conditions that one should try to match are: alveolar ventilation, cardiac output, $\dot{V}O_2$ and FiO_2. To the extent that those conditions cannot be matched, some knowledge of how much such factors can affect the calculated venous admixture would be useful. This requires theoretical calculations of the type reported by West (1). Figure 1, taken from this work, gives an isolated example of the potential importance of this problem in a lung containing a moderate but not severe degree of $\dot{V}_A/\dot{Q}$ mismatch breathing room air. Venous admixture is seen to vary from about 36 to about 6% as alveolar ventilaton is increased from 4 to 12 L/min. West's algorithm, recently updated (5) to increase efficiency, is well suited to such calculations, allowing a wide range of conditions to be studied.

Importance of knowing mixed venous PO_2 in gas exchange analysis

While bound up in the above comments, it is worth separately stressing how important a knowledge of mixed venous PO_2 is when caculating venous admixture. Figures 2A and 2B demonstrate how the calculation of venous admixture yields very different results depending on whether $P\bar{v}O_2$ is assumed (A) or measured (B). In A, $P\bar{v}O_2$ is assumed to result in an arteriovenous O_2 content difference of 5 ml/100 ml, while in B, $P\bar{v}O_2$ rises as cardiac output rises to maintain $\dot{V}O_2$ at constant levels. Condition B is more appropriate to reality, with meta-

144

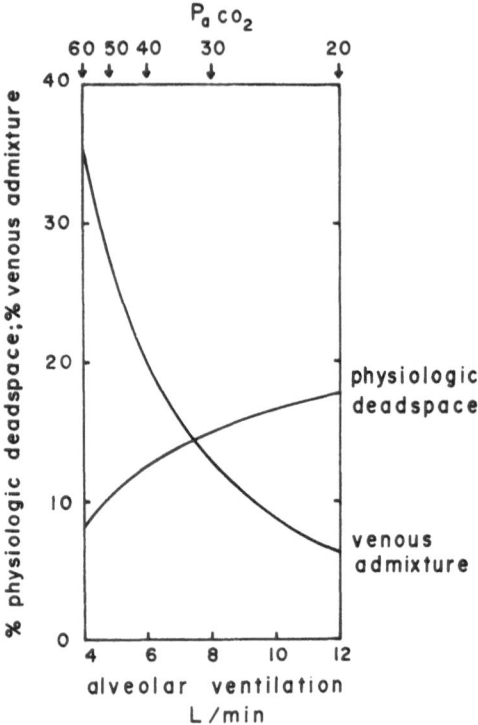

Figure 1. Dependence of physiologic dead space and venous admixture on alveolar ventilation in a theoretical lung model with a fixed degree of moderately severe $\dot{V}_A/\dot{Q}$ mismatching. Notice how at different levels of ventilation these two indices are considerably dependent upon overall alveolar ventilation. Similar dependency is noted for variation in cardiac output, but as cardiac output rises, venous admixture rises and physiologic dead space falls. Arterial PCO_2 values corresponding to each level of alveolar ventilation are indicated at the top.

bolic rate constant. These curves demonstrate for two hypothetical patients how important the assumption of $P\bar{v}O_2$ is. Patient A has a 25% shunt but no $\dot{V}_A/\dot{Q}$ mismatch, while Patient B has only $\dot{V}_A/\dot{Q}$ mismatch. Both are breathing 40% inspired O_2. Thus, assuming a constant arteriovenous difference would result in an apparent fall in venous admixture for 35 to 20% as cardiac output increases from 4 to 8 L/min in Patient A, when in fact, there was no change in venous admixture. However, if mixed venous PO_2 had been measured and used as in Figure 2B, the correct of value of venous admixture would have been calculated at all cardiac output levels. While not strictly true for Patient B, it is evident that in this particular example, venous admixture is not sensitive to cardiac output when mixed venous PO_2 is known (Figure 2B), although large errors occur if $P\bar{v}O_2$ is assumed (Figure 2A). The difficulty in making general quantitative statements about this problem in the presence of $\dot{V}_A/\dot{Q}$ mismatch is evident in comparing Figures 1 and 2B where effects of ventilation and cardiac output on venous admixture are shown for two lungs with similar degrees of $\dot{V}_A/\dot{Q}$ mis-

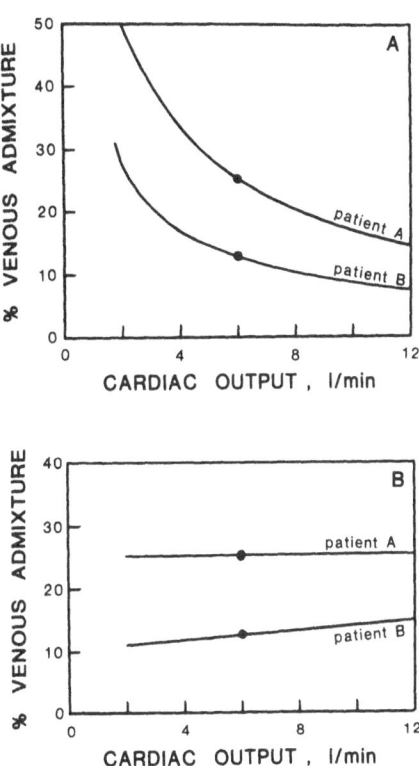

Figure 2. Dependence of venous admixture on cardiac output in two hypothetical patients. For details of the patients, see text. In panel A, venous admixture is calculated assuming a constant arteriovenous O_2 content difference of 5 vol %. In panel B, venous admixture was calculated from the correct arteriovenous O_2 content differences (which vary inversely with cardiac output). In Patient A, with a pure shunt, assumption of mixed venous PO_2 will lead to large errors if the cardiac output is different from the assumed value. Similar effects are noted for Patient B, who has $\dot{V}_A/\dot{Q}$ mismatching. Knowledge of the true mixed venous PO_2 eliminates the dependence of venous admixture on cardiac output in the case of a true shunt, and reduces it in the presence of $\dot{V}_A/\dot{Q}$ inequality.

match. The difference is simply that $FiO_2 = 0.21$ in Figure 1 and 0.4 in Figure 2B, placing the lung unit endcapillary PO_2 values on different parts of the O_2 dissocia-tion curve. Consequently, without some way of knowing the quantitative features of the $\dot{V}_A/\dot{Q}$ distribution and of carrying out the calculations discussed here, there remains a difficult problem interpreting changes in venous admixture when extrapulmonary factors change.

Influence of cardiac output on PaO_2

The effects that changes in cardiac output have on one's ability to interpret PaO_2 were discussed above. This section will illustrate this from a different viewpoint by the comparison of two actual patients whose PaO_2 values were very different.

146

Patient A is asthmatic and had a PaO$_2$ of 84 Torr. Patient B was in pulmonary edema following a myocardial infarct and had a PaO$_2$ of 55 Torr. We measured their distributions of $\dot{V}_A/\dot{Q}$ by multiple inert gas elimination (6, 7, 8) and the results appear in Figure 3A (asthma) and 3B (myocardial infarct). What can be seen from Figure 3 is that the asthmatic patient has about 20% of the cardiac output associated with low $\dot{V}_A/\dot{Q}$ areas of very low alveolar PO$_2$ while the patient with edema has only about 13% of the cardiac output associated with zero or low

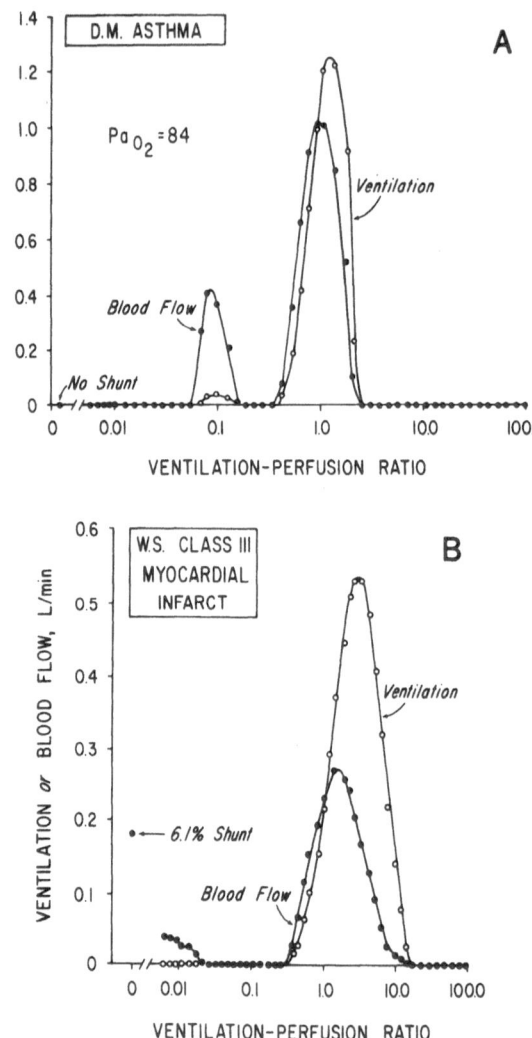

Figure 3. Distributions of ventilation–perfusion ratios in a patient with asthma (A) and a patient in pulmonary edema following a myocardial infarct (B). The asthmatic subject has more $\dot{V}_A/\dot{Q}$ mismatch with about 20% of the cardiac output associated with very low $\dot{V}_A/\dot{Q}$ areas. The patient following myocardial infarction has only 13% of the cardic output associated with poorly or unventilated areas, yet his arterial PO$_2$ was 55 Torr, compared to the asthmatic's of 84 Torr. The reason why arterial PO$_2$ is higher in the presence of more $\dot{V}_A/\dot{Q}$ mismatching in the asthmatic subject is the much higher value of cardiac output.

$\dot{V}_A/\dot{Q}$ areas. This would at first sight lead one to expect that the edematous patient would have the higher PaO_2 due to lesser $\dot{V}_A/\dot{Q}$ mismatch, but in fact the opposite was true. The explanation was that the asthmatic patient had a cardiac output of 7 L/min and a mixed venous PO_2 of 40 Torr, while the edematous patient, due to the myocardial infarct, had a cardiac output of only 2.5 L/min and a mixed venous PO_2 of 23 Torr. These two patients graphically demonstrate that more $\dot{V}_A/\dot{Q}$ inequality does not necessarily result in more severe hypoxemia, and that differences in cardiac output can considerably affect PaO_2.

FiO$_2$ and quantification of gas exchange abnormality

Inspired PO_2 is one extrapulmonary factor that clearly has a major influence on arterial PO_2, and, in the presence of $\dot{V}_A/\dot{Q}$ mismatch, a major effect on venous admixture values even when mixed venous PO_2 has been measured and used in the calculations. In the clinical case of critically ill patients, therefore, evaluation of gas exchange must take account of FiO_2. It is difficult to do this if FiO_2 is changed and so one custom has been to carry out such evaluations at different times at a constant FiO_2. This section comments on the choice of FiO_2 at which such evaluations should be made.

Because most critically ill patients have poorly ventilated areas of low $\dot{V}_A/\dot{Q}$ venous admixture will progressively fall as FiO_2 is raised until at $FiO_2 = 1.0$, venous admixture will reflect only true shunt. Therefore it seems rational that in order to estimate as much of the abnormality as possible, the evaluation should be carried out at the *lowest* rather than *highest* FiO_2 attainable. Realistically, patients are ventilated with gas whose FiO_2 is usually above that of room air because lower values of FiO_2 result in unacceptable hypoxemia. Thus, the lowest FiO_2 attainable is suggested as being the maintenance value with which the patient is being treated, rather than some lower value that would endanger the patient.

Such a choice will uncover the greatest degree of $\dot{V}_A/\dot{Q}$ mismatch safely attainable by PO_2 measurement, and this gives a more accurate picture of the total pulmonary gas exchange state than measurement at higher FiO_2 values.

However, there are other distinct advantages of this choice. One is practical. Whenever FiO_2 is altered, it takes 15 min to 1 hr to reach steady-state conditions before meaningful measurements can be obtained. This wastes time and money, both of which can be avoided if the patient is evaluated at his maintenance FiO_2. Another reason is that elevating the inspired PO_2 may well worsen the $\dot{V}_A/\dot{Q}$ distribution both by releasing hypoxic vasoconstriction in previously hypoxic low $\dot{V}_A/\dot{Q}$ areas (which will increase their perfusion) and by promoting absorption atelectasis (9, 10). Such changes will worsen the functional state of the lungs to the possible detriment of the patient and cause larger estimates of abnormality to be calculated that existed at the lower maintenance FiO_2. Hence, the recommendation is made that gas exchange be evaluated at the maintenance FiO_2 of the patient.

GAS EXCHANGE DURING HIGH-FREQUENCY OSICLLATORY VENTILATION (HFOV)

All of the principles discussed above apply to HFOV, but there are some special considerations in addition. Table 1 shows the issues that will be dealt with in this chapter. However, in every case, while some data appear in the literature, more work will be required to fully understand how HFOV permits adequate gas exchange and affects mucociliary transport. Not all frequencies have been explored, nor are there enough published data to make clear-cut general statements. Thus the conclusions reached herein should be considered as current but subject to change as more experience is gained with HFOV. The choice of topics covered in this section is made to reflect the author's experience and also so as not to overlap significantly with the chapter by Dr A.C. Bryan in this volume.

Efficacy of HFOV in the presence of intrapulmonary shunting

High-frequency ventilation has been shown to be effective in maintaining gas exchange in the presence of shunting (11, 12). These studies were of oleic acid-induced hemorrhagic pulmonary edema in dogs and rabbits, and whether the results will apply to human pulmonary edema is not clear. This is because dogs have a more compliant chest wall than adult man, and also because oleic acid-induced edema is frankly hemorrhagic and is unlike common forms of edema in man. Thompon's study (12) suggests that the efficacy of HFOV in this setting is mediated through its PEEP-like effect on alveolar pressure and hence lung volume. If this is true, then there may be no basic difference in effectiveness between HFOV and conventional ventilation - both appear to exert their beneficial effect on gas exchange via expansion of edematous/atelectatic areas and thus the potential for barotrauma and cardiac output depression may be similar.

Bryan has presented evidence (13) relating efficacy of HFOV in infants with respiratory distress to lung volume history. Thus, if the lungs are ventilated with HFOV after an inflation, oxygenation is much better than HFOV at a similar mean pressure, but without prior inflation. This makes sense in terms of the well-known hysteresis of the lung pressure volume curve in that lung volume will be higher after the inflation. It would appear from these results that HFOV can maintain oxygenation in edematous lungs, but periodic hyperinflation may be an important maneuver to use to prevent atelectasis.

Efficacy of HFOV in the presence of ventilation/perfusion inequality

While it seems that HFOV can maintain gas exchange when units are previously unventilated if alveolar pressures are raised enough to have a PEEP-like effect, the issue of whether HFOV is effective in the presence of airway obstruction is an entirely different matter. Here, alveoli are usually expanded and often normal, and it is the airways that, because of obstruction with mucus, mucosal edema or bronchoconstriction, prevent adequate distal ventilation.

One could predict that HFOV might have a special advantage over conventional ventilation in this setting. This prediction is based on the supposition that at low frequencies, resistive impedance to airflow is governed by Poiseuille's law and therefore flow is proportional to the 4th power of the radius. However, at high frequencies, the inertial component of impedance will become increasingly important as a factor governing ventilation. It turns out that as discussed by Banzett and Lehr (14), inertial impedance is inversely related to the 2nd power of the airway radius, such that ventilation becomes proportional to radius squared when this component dominates. To the extent that this simple hypothesis holds under in vivo conditions, one would predict that in the presence of a nonuniform distribution of airway diameters, as is characteristic of all obstructive diseases, the distribution of ventilation would be more even during HFOV than conventional ventilaton.

This hypothesis would have major therapeutic implications if borne out by experimental work. Preliminary results carried out in a simple two 'alveolus' physical model and also in an isolated dog lung with left main bronchus luminal obstruction do support this hypothesis (15), at least at 10–20 Hz. The effect is only seen in severe obstruction (i.e. when the diameter of the left main bronchus is reduced by a factor of 10 or so), but under such conditions, the ratio of left to right lung ventilation is about 5 times greater than with conventional ventilation.

Taken to the intact dog, however, additional factors may well have to be considered. Thus it is increasingly evident that alveolar pressures are considerably higher than mean airway pressures largely due to the Bernoulli effect. Consequently, lung volume is higher than expected. This phenomenon may well occur differently behind a normal airway compared to an obstructed airway. If there is more alveolar expansion distal to the normal airways, this would have a PEEP-like effect in diverting blood flow away from the normal to the poorly ventilated areas. Such an effect will give rise to less efficient gas exchange so that the potential benefit of HFOV in better ventilating obstructed units may be outweighed by the disadvantage of redistribution of perfusion. While there is preliminary data (15, 16) on the efficacy of HFOV in the presence of airway obstructions, suggesting that *overall* there is little difference between it and conventional ventilation with respect to gas exchange, much more work needs to be done before firm conclusions can be drawn. However, what can be concluded now is that there is no substantial overall advantage to HFDV in the presence of airway obstructions (with inflated alveoli distal to the obstruction).

Mucociliary clearance and gas exchange

During conventional ventilation, mucus secretion and mucociliary clearance have been shown to be of great importance in gas exchange. Mucus plugging in asthma and airway secretions in chronic bronchitis are widely known to be associated with poor distal alveolar ventilation and hence hypoxemia. Consequently, any effect HFOV has on mucus secretion and mucociliary clearance has major implications for gas exchange. There is anecdotal evidence that patients put on HFOV rapidly present copius secretions at the trachea. The implication is that HFOV promotes mucociliary clearance and this is seen as a positive benefit of HFOV. However, another interpretation is possible – the secretions seen in the uper airways might be locally produced in response to the irritation of rapid airway diameter changes plus the high sheer stresses of rapid gas flow along the airway wall caused by HFOV. Clearly, measurement of mucociliary function must be made before conclusions can be drawn. McEvoy et al. (17) measured clearance of deposited radioactive aerosol during HFOV and found it to be completely inhibited throughout a 4 hr period of HFOV (Figure 4), while during mechanical ventilaton clearance was observed. At the same time, considerable tracheal mucus was observed bronchoscopically, consistent with the anecdotes cited above. These findings suggest that the upper airway mucus is locally produced probably in response to airway irritation. Further, the inhibition of clearance must be viewed as a negative effect of HFOV that could be highly significant for patients with airway secretions. McEvoy's results were obtained at a single frequency of 20 Hz only, and recently rapid chest wall compression at lower frequencies was found to enhance tracheal mucus velocity (18). Whether

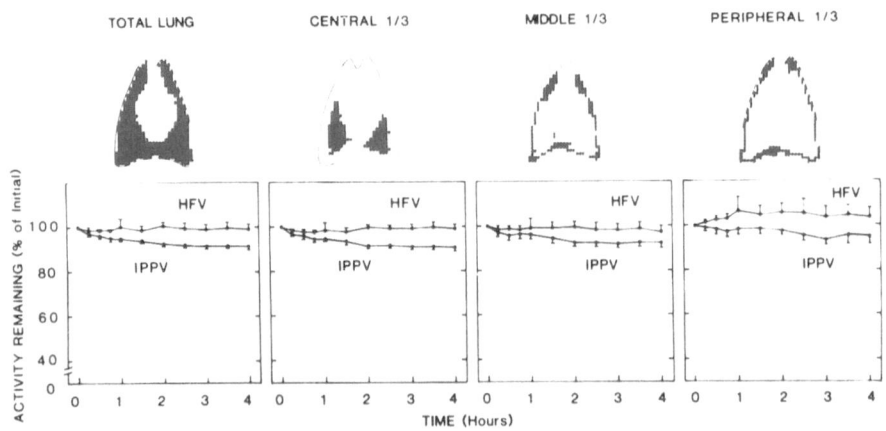

Figure 4. Mucociliary clearance as detected by external counting of previously deposited radioactive aerosol in normal dogs. During high-frequency ventilation, clearance is completely inhibited, whereas during conventional mechanical ventilation (IPPV), gradual clearance is observed over 4 hr.

this difference is due to the chest wall compression (rather than airway oscillatory ventilation) or to the lower frequencies, remains to be determined.

In any event, the effects of any form of high-frequency ventilation on mucus secretion and on mucociliary clearance must be studied in detail before the safety and efficacy of HFV can be completely established.

ACKNOWLEDGEMENT

This work was supported by NIH Grant HL-17731, and I wish to thank Tania Davisson for her assistance in the preparation of this paper.

REFERENCES

1. West JB: Ventilation–perfusion inequality and overall gas exchange in computer models of the lung. Respir Physiol 7:88–110, 1969
2. Wagner PD: Ventilation–perfusion inequality in catastrophic lung disease. In: Prakash O (ed), Applied Physiology in Clinical Respiratory Care. Martinus Nijhoff, The Hague/Boston/London, pp 363–379, 1982
3. Pontoppidan H, Geffin B, Lowenstein E: Acute Respiratory Failure in the Adult. Little, Brown & Co, Boston, 1973
4. Rahn H, Fenn WO: In: A Graphical Analysis of the Respiratory Gas Exchange. Am Physio Soc, Washington, DC, 1955
5. West JB, Wagner PD: Pulmonary gas exchange. In: West JB (ed), Bioengineering Aspects of the Lung. Marcel Dekker, New York, 1977
6. Wagner PD, Naumann PF, Laravuso RB: Simultaneous measurement of eight foreign gases in blood by gas chromatography. J Appl Physiol 36:600–605, 1974
7. Wagner PD, Laravuso RB, Uhl RR, West JB: Continuous distributions of ventilation–perfusion ratios in normal subjects breathing air and 100% O_2. J Clin Invest 54:54–68, 1974
8. Evans JW, Wagner PD: Limits on $\dot{V}_A/\dot{Q}$ distributions from analysis of experimental inert gas eliminations. J Appl Physiol 42:899–898, 1977
9. Briscoe WA, Cree EM, Filler S, Houssay HEJ, Cournand A: Lung volume, alveolar ventilation and perfusion interrelationships in chronic pulmonary emphysema. J Appl Physiol 15:785–795, 1960
10. Dantzker DR, Wagner PD, West JB: Instability of lung units with low $\dot{V}_A/\dot{Q}$ ratios during O_2 breathing. J Appl Physiol 38:886–895, 1975
11. Wright K, Lyrene RK, Truog WE, Standaert TA, Murphy J, Woodrum DE: Ventilation by high-frequency oscillation in rabbits with oleic acid lung disease. J Appl Physiol 50:1056–1060, 1981
12. Thompson WK, Marchak BE, Froese AB, Bryan AC: High-frequency oscillation compared with standard ventilation in pulmonary injury model. J Appl Physiol 52:543–548, 1982
13. Bryan AC: Volume history effect of HFOV on PO_2. Report of Workshop on High-Frequency Ventilation, New Orleans, Louisiana, December 5–7, 1982
14. Banzett RB, Lehr JL: Gas exchange during high-frequency ventilation of the chicken. J Appl Physiol 53:1418–1422, 1982
15. Koga H, Wagner PD: Distribution of ventilation in isolated lungs with airway obstruction during high-frequency ventilation. Fed Proc (abstract) (in press)
16. Kaiser KG, Davies NJH, Rodriguez-Roisin R, Bencowitz HZ, Wagner PD: Efficiency of high-

frequency ventilation in the presence of extensive ventilation/perfusion mismatching. Am Rev Respir Dis 124:233, 1979

17. McEvoy RD, Davies NJH, Hedenstierna G, Hartman MT, Spragg RG, Wagner PD: Lung mucociliary transport during high-frequency ventilation. Am Rev Respir Dis 126:452–456, 1981

18. King M, Phillips DM, Gross D, Vartian V, Chang HK, Zidulka A: Enhanced tracheal mucus clearance with high-frequency chest wall compression. Am Rev Respir Dis 128:511–515, 1983

14. HOME OXYGEN IN INFANTS WITH CHRONIC LUNG DISEASE

HEATHER BRYAN, A.L. CAMPBELL, Y. ZARFIN and M. GROENVELD

INTRODUCTION

Over the past decade the survival of prematurely born infants has steadily risen (1). Many of these infants however have respiratory insufficiency, either bronchopulmonary dysplasia (BPD) or Wilson-Mikity syndrome, and require supplementary oxygen therapy for weeks to several months after birth (2, 3). Conventional methods of administering oxygen to babies in incubators or in head hoods does not allow for a close physical relationship between the infants and their parents. Normal procedures such as feeding, bathing, holding and cuddling are delayed and this may affect the development and behavior of these infants. The delivery of oxygen through a nasal tube was introduced in infants by Pinney et al. in 1976 (4). With this method the infant is cared for in an open bassinet, and can be held, bathed, and 'mothered', as well as breast or bottle fed without interfering with oxygen delivery. Infants are now being discharged home on nasal oxygen therapy under the care of their families and this report summarizes the experience at a large urban hospital over a three-year period.

METHODS

Nasal catheter oxygen system

Oxygen is delivered through a feeding cathether (8FG) inserted approximately one centimeter into one nostril and secured by tape to the upper lip and malar area (Figure 1A). The oxygen given is not mixed with air, but is delivered at a concentration of 100% from a wall or cylinder source at a low-flow rate via a low-flow meter (0–2 L) and O_2 tubing to the nasal catheter. Conventional pediatric wall flow meters (0–15 L) do not allow a fine enough adjustment at the low flows used (up to 500 ml/min). The oxygen flow rate requirement is determined individually in each infant using transcutaneous oxygen tension ($tcPO_2$) monitoring over 1–2 hr of sleep (5). The rate is adjusted to maintain a stable $tcPO_2$ reading of >50 mmHg and <80 mmHg during sleep and two hours is essential to include

154

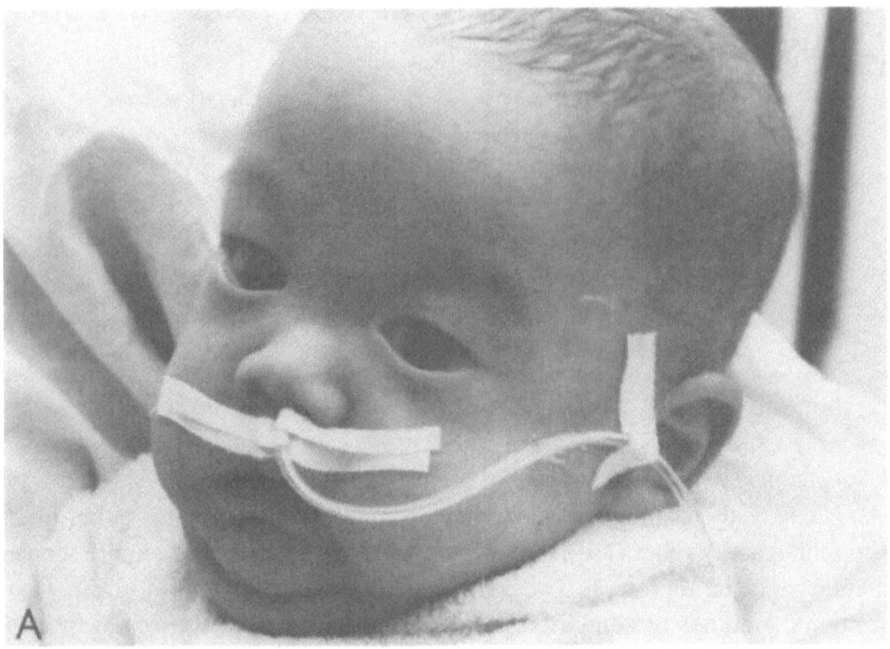

Figure 1. Low-flow oxygen delivered to an infant either through a secured nasal catheter (A) or a soft rubber catheter lying across the upper lip with 2 holes positioned at the nares (B). ⟶

quiet, REM and indeterminant sleep states. Several 2-hr studies are done to assure a stable oxygen intake has been achieved. This method allows the infant to breathe room air along with the 100% low-flow oxygen, the mixing occurring in the nasal passages and upper pharynx. Because minute ventilation varies in each infant, the actual concentration of inspired oxygen can only be approximated.

In order to allow easy handling of the infant the O_2 tubing is 15 to 30 feet in length and connections to the low-flow meter and the nasal catheter must be secure. A pressure manometer introduced into the circuit line indicates a continuous oxygen flow (low-pressure reading), an obstruction (elevated pressure reading) or a break in the line (no flow) (Figure 2). In the home cylinder O_2 is used as the source, and the family provided with a large capacity size and a small portable cylinder (Figure 2).

Selection of infants

Stable babies requiring inspired oxygen concentrations of less than 50% and who weigh more than 1600 grams are placed on low-flow, nasal catheter oxygen in the neonatal nursery. Smaller infants are unsuitable as the nasal catheter (8F) may

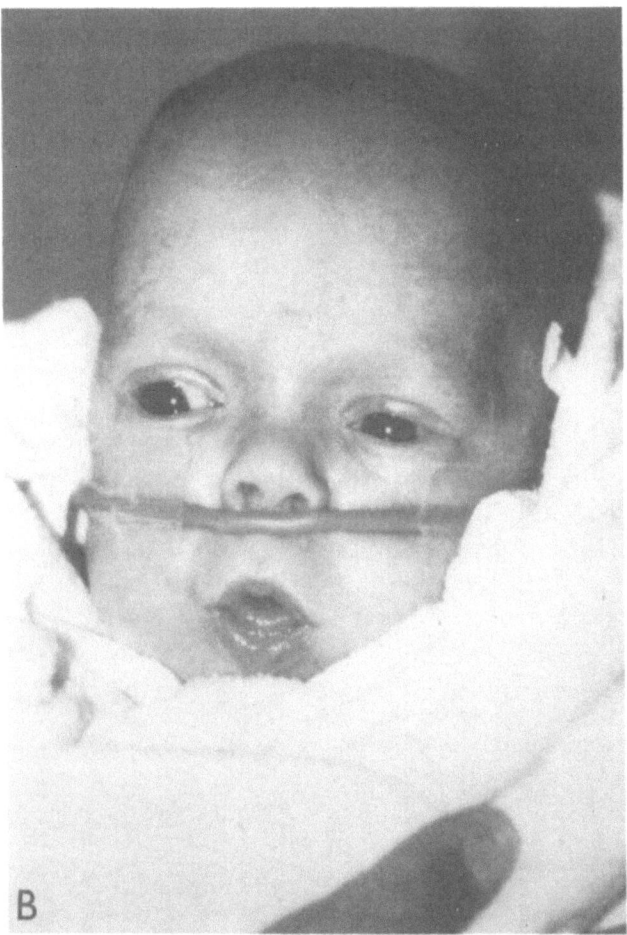

block an entire nostril while smaller sized catheters offer too much resistance to flow making it unsafe to ensure a continuous circuit.

Recently soft rubber gavage (urethral) catheters (10F) placed across the upper lip, rather than into the nostril have been used successfully in infants weighing more than 1000 grams requiring less than 35% O_2. The end-hole is covered with tape and two holes cut in the catheter and positioned at the nares (Figure 1B). The additional advantage of this noninvasive technique is fewer changes and less blocking with nasal secretions.

Once oxygen requirements are established the babies are monitored in hospital by $tcPO_2$ 2 to 3 times per week. In older infants with chronic lung disease, bronchopulmonary dysplasia (BPD) or Wilson-Mikity syndrome, oxygen requirements usually remain stable for 2 to 4 weeks and it was this finding which led to the suggestion of discharge on home oxygen.

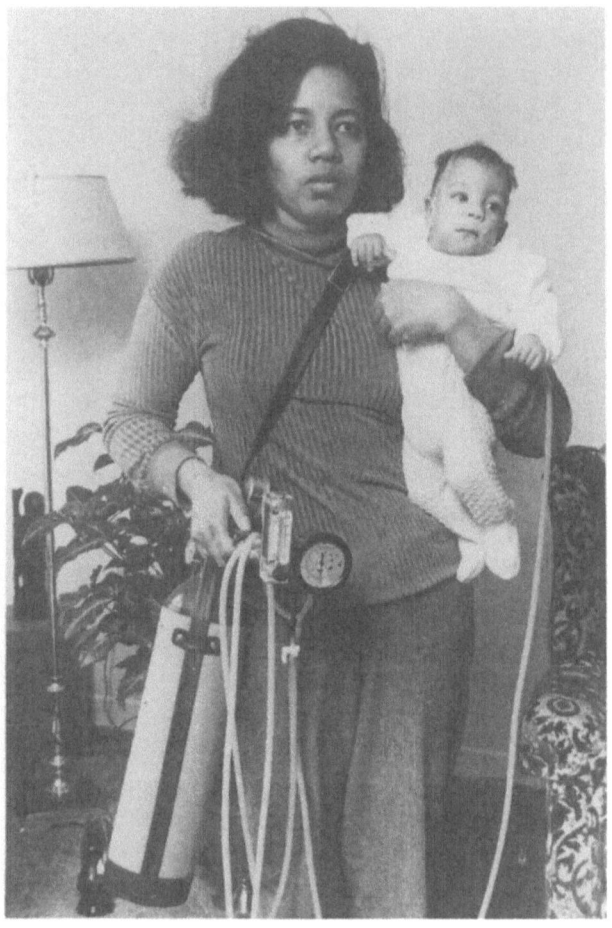

Figure 2. The portable oxygen cylinder, low-flow oxygen meter, pressure manometer, delivery tubing and infant on LFO$_2$ shown with mother at home.

Discharge criteria

Infants are discharged home if they weigh >2500 grams and are medically stable on low-flow O$_2$. In addition other important discharge criteria include complete acceptance by the parents, a family physician/pediatrician willing to assist in the home program, a satisfactory assessment of the home by a Public Health nurse, and a home with more than one resident adult. Where these latter criteria cannot be met then the infant is transferred to the nearest local childrens hospital, or to a pediatric convalescent hospital.

Training of parents

A two-week training program for the parents is given by the ward nurses and respiratory technologists to ensure competence and complete understanding of the low-flow technique. In addition parents are carefully instructed in the symptoms of hypoxia (cyanosis, tachypnea, apnea, or signs of respiratory infection) so that if these occur at home, immediate medical advice is sought and prompt admission to hospital is organized.

Reassessment

Infants are readmitted to hospital monthly for 48 to 72 hr to reassess and adjust with tcPO$_2$ monitoring the low-flow oxygen requirements.

RESULTS

Forty-six infants were discharged over a 3-year period on LFO$_2$ on ranges of 0.05 to 0.5 L/min. Twenty (43%) of these infants lived outside the urban center up to a distance of 1800 km. Twenty-nine were discharged home and nineteen to their local hospitals. The respiratory illnesses and clinical details are shown in Table 1. Bronchopulmonary dysplasia was the commonest lung condition ($n = 38$), while 8 infants had Wilson-Mikity syndrome. The age of discharge and age of cessation of LFO$_2$ are shown in Table 2.

Of those twenty-nine infants discharged home, one was readmitted 4 days later because the family failed in management, and twenty-eight infants were suc-

Table 1. Infants treated with low-flow oxygen (LFO$_2$).

	Bronchopulmonary dysplasia $n = 38$ mean (range)	Wilson-Mikity syndrome $n = 8$ mean (range)
Gestation (wks)	30.2 (24–37)	28.3 (27–31)
Birth weight (kg)	1.28 (0.6–2.3)	1.17 (0.7–1.5)
IPPV (days)	16 (2–76)	2 (0–7)
CPAP (days)	7 (0–30)	4 (0–17)
Isolette O$_2$ (days)	44 (2–134)	43 (21–68)

158

Table 2. Low-flow oxygen (LFO$_2$) treatment.

	Bronchopulmonary dysplasia $n = 38$ Age (wks) mean (range)	Wilson-Mikity syndrome $n = 8$ Age (wks) mean (range)
Home on LFO$_2$	18.1 (5–59)	15.3 (9–25)
Off LFO$_2$	29.9 (9–75)	29.3 (15–45)

cessfully weaned from LFO$_2$. The shortest duration of home therapy was 9 weeks while the longest was 9 months. One 15-month old infant with severe BPD went home on LFO$_2$ for 4 months, but died shortly after readmission to hospital with severe bronchopneumonia. One infant aged 9 months died suddenly at home 9 days after LFO$_2$ therapy was discontinued. The postmortem diagnosis showed residual BPD and bronchopneumonia. A second infant, aged 5 months, also died suddenly at home 6 weeks after home oxygen was discontinued. The postmortem showed Wilson-Mikity syndrome. All the 19 infants referred to local hospitals were weaned from LFO$_2$ and all survived. Eight infants were readmitted to hospital during the home O$_2$ therapy for management of respiratory infections on 12 separate occasions. None of the 46 infants developed retrolental fibroplasia while on the LFO$_2$ program.

For those infants who were treated with LFO$_2$ at home the cost for in-hospital treatment was $ 156 per day. The total number of days for the 29 infants treated at home was 2287, correcting for readmissions for respiratory illnesses and the monthly in-hospital reassessments. This comprises a financial saving of approximately $ 350 000 or $ 12 000 per infant. In contrast the cost for supplies at home (O$_2$, nasal catheters, etc.) was $ 100 per month per baby.

DISCUSSION

Treating stable infants who are oxygen dependent in a home environment allows for more normal infant/parent contacts, enhancing family relationships. The LFO$_2$ method itself has been shown to achieve a more stable oxygen delivery when compared to O$_2$ delivered into a hood or incubator (5) and improved weight gain has also been demonstrated (6).

Home oxygen management does entail some risk for the infant. One of our infants with severe BPD and respiratory failure died in hospital at 19 months of age. This death was expected by ourselves and the parents. Two infants with residual chronic lung disease, however, died suddenly at home after the home oxygen treatment was terminated at 9 days and 6 weeks. Since the occurrence of these deaths infants now remain on home apnea monitors for two months after the home oxygen therapy.

It is important that the parents are enthusiastic about the home oxygen program. If they are not, then the babies remain in hospitals as near to the home as possible. None of our parents wished to abandon the program once it started, although one family failed in the management. Many families, however, were grateful for the monthly readmissions of 2–3 days for reassessment as these periods allowed families a respite from the constant vigilance needed in looking after an oxygen-dependent infant. It is because of these demands that two adults must live in the home in order to share the burden of responsibility. The importance of repeated and careful training of parents in hospital prior to the infants discharge cannot be overemphasized.

The introduction of oxygen delivery by a catheter across the upper lip (Figure 1B) rather than the nasal route, makes the home management easier. Portable oxygen packs have also allowed more freedom at home, including transport by car, descreasing the need for ambulance transfer, and in allowing the family short trips from home for pleasure outings.

The costs of maintaining oxygen in the home, including supplies, etc., was approximately $ 100 per month compared to $ 12 000 per infant if hospital care had continued until the babies were off supplemental oxygen. The benefits to any Health Care Program, whether national or individual, are obvious.

REFERENCES

1. Hack M, Fanaroff AA, Merkatz IR: The low birth weight infant – evolution of a changing outlook. N Engl J Med 301:1162–1165, 1979
2. Bancalari E, Abdenour GE, Feller R, Gannon J: Bronchopulmonary dysplasia: clinical presentation. J Pediatr 95: 819–823, 1979
3. Wung JT, Koons AH, Driscoll JM Jr, James LS: Changing incidence of bronchopulmonary dysplasia. 95:845–847, 1979
4. Pinney MA, Cotton EK: Home management of bronchopulmonary dysplasia. J Pediatr 58:856–859, 1976
5. Philip AGS, Peadbody JL, Lucey JF: Transcutaneous PO_2 monitoring in the home management of bronchopulmonary dysplasia. Pediatrics 61:655–657, 1978
6. Cox MA, Cohen AJ, Slavin RF, Epstein MF: Improved growth in infants with bronchopulmonary dysplasia treated with nasal cannula oxygen. Pediatr Res 13:1001, 1979

15. HOME MONITORING IN SIDS

Heather Bryan and Paul Duffty

INTRODUCTION

Over the past decade a great deal of attention has been focused on the sudden infant death syndrome (SIDS), the leading cause of death in infants between the ages of 1 to 12 months. During the last 20 years of investigation and research, hypotheses have abounded in attempting to understand why a well baby dies suddenly without conclusive postmortem evidence of lethal disease. The literature contains many theories including infection, metabolic deficiencies or excesses, immunological reactions, endocrine or neurological problems, all investigated and found wanting (1). The list continues to be added to, so that we have a 'Theory of the Month Club', often intemperate and pseudoscientific, leading to intense medical controversy, as well as media pressure on anxious parents and doctors.

What is known is that well infants die silently while asleep, the majority occurring between ages 2 to 5 months. In approximately one half of the cases there has been a mild upper respiratory tract infection 5 to 10 days before death. Premature infants, siblings of SIDS victims and infants from multiple births are at a higher risk than the random incidence of 1 to 3 deaths per 1000 live births (1). These epidemiological facts suggest that it is improbable that there is a single cause of SIDS.

Special pathological studies have demonstrated that 50–60% of SIDS infants have tissue changes consistent with chronic hypoxia or oxygen lack (2, 3). These changes are exactly the same as those demonstrated in babies dying of chronic lung disease or cyanotic structural heart anomalies. However as the heart and lungs in SIDS victims are normal, the data suggests that there is a failure in the control of respiration and breathing is inadequate to meet metabolic needs. This failure can be explained either by the occurrence of repeated apneic episodes or hypoventilation, both of which can lead to significant hypoxia. In order to investigate these possibilities infant sleep laboratories were instituted to examine normal and high risk infants. Because sleep is not a homogeneous state, sophisticated and costly monitoring is required. Recordings of EEG, eye movements and skeletal muscle tone are done to distinguish sleep state, along with respiration measured in a variety of ways, and also cardiac function by recording heart rate.

The most difficult parameter to measure is tidal volume or the amount of air inspired each breath over hours of sleep. The technology has not been available and all reports to date include only respiratory frequency. Nor have researchers been able to measure arterial oxygenation in order to know whether enough oxygen is reaching the tissues. Transcutaneous monitoring although widely used on sick infants in neonatal intensive care units, is not satisfactory in older normal infants during prolongued sleep studies.

Without these two important measurements of respiratory volume or tissue oxygenation, the reports from infant sleep laboratories have found little to distinguish infants at risk for SIDS from normal babies (4). Certainly the investigators have not been able to find a predictive test for SIDS. Apneic pauses of unusual length (>20 seconds) have not been commonly reported. Periodic breathing, a cyclical respiratory pattern common to early infancy has been reported to occur more commonly in siblings of SIDS infants by one group of investigators (5), but the reverse is seen by another (6). Obstructive apnea, where respiratory movements are seen, but no air enters the lungs because of upper airway closure caused by relaxation of the muscles controlling the tongue, jaw and pharynx, has not been a prominent feature seen during high risk infant sleep studies (7).

The cause or causes of SIDS therefore remain obscure despite many concerted and costly investigations carried out over the past decade. What do we do then with high risk infants while researchers strive to find a cause? Our hospital has been one of several centers to use home electronic monitors in an effort to prevent death from SIDS and our nine-year experience is related in this report.

SUBJECTS AND METHODS

Infants referred to the hospital from 1974–1982 following episodes of apparent 'lifelessness' at home entered the home monitor program only if no treatable cause was found during an extensive medical investigation (8). There were 124 of these near-miss infants, all but 19 of whom were fullterm at birth. Also enrolled in the home monitor program were 126 siblings of SIDS infants, 15 of whom were premature at birth. Thirteen of these infants were referred because of an apnea spell, and 10 were survivors from 9 multiple births, all associated with a SIDS death.

The infants were placed on the home monitor for at least one night, to test the reliability of the monitor in hospital. The parents were instructed by the nursing staff on at least two occasions in the use of the monitor and in methods of resuscitation (Table 1). They were also interviewed by one of the physicians associated with the home monitor program and asked to keep a record of any spells which occurred, and also to record false alarms. The parents were con-

Table 1. Methods of resuscitation.

---

1. Tactile stimulation
2. Arousal
3. Cardiopulmonary

---

tacted at least once a month by telephone. We supervised the home monitor program only and were not the family's primary physician.

The home monitor used depended on availability and included the transducer-pad type (Electronic Monitors Inc., model RE134 C or D, Fort Worth, Texas) in 185 infants; heart rate monitors (Parks Manufacturing Inc., model 510A, Beaverton, Oregon) in 42 infants, and 23 infant chest impedance monitors (Air Shields, model Am-46-1, Hatboro, Pennsylvania). The monitors were set to alarm for nonbreathing pauses of 20 sec or heart rates less than 60 beats per minute. Monitoring continued at home until the babies had no spells for two months or in the SIDS siblings without apnea, until 6 months of age.

RESULTS

Fourteen near-miss infants presented with a life-threatening spell observed in hospital during the first 7 days of life. None of these infants had any further apnea/bradycardia on their home monitors, and monitoring was discontinued at 3.5 ± 2.3 months (mean ± 1SD).

Of the 110 remaining infants, 63 (57%) had no further spells at home, while 47 (43%) did (Table 2). Ninety-nine (90%) of the near-miss infants started home monitoring during the first four months of age. The mean ages for placement on and for coming off the home monitors for the 2 groups is shown in Table 2.

Table 2. Home monitoring.

	n	Age on monitor (months)[a]	Age off monitor (months)[a]	Total time on monitor (months)[a]	Death on monitor n
Near-miss					
Spells at home	47	2.3 ± 1.4	10.9 ± 3.8	8.6 ± 3.8	0
No spells at home	63	2.7 ± 1.7	6.5 ± 2.4	3.7 ± 2.4	0
SIDS siblings					
Spells at home	43	1.3 ± 2.1	9.2 ± 3.1	8.1 ± 2.5	1
No spells at home	83	1.3 ± 2.1	7.2 ± 2.2	6.4 ± 2.1	1

[a] mean ± 1SD

Thirteen of the infants with apnea/bradycardiac spells were on home monitoring longer than 12 months of age. Resuscitation used during a spell included tactile stimulation and/or arousal in all but two instances. All of the infants have survived.

Spells on the home monitor occurred in 45 SIDS siblings, less commonly (34%) than in the near-miss group. Ninety-eight infants (78%) entered the program during the first month of life. The mean ages on and off the home monitors are shown in Table 2. Only 9 infants remained on the monitor for longer than the first year of life. Again, as with the near-miss group of infants, those who had spells were resuscitated mainly by stimulation and/or arousal. Two infants, however, were found profoundly pale and apneic by their mothers when the monitors alarmed, and both were given cardiopulmonary resuscitation. Although both infants were taken to hospital by ambulance with continuing oxygen and re-suscitation therapy, neither survived. One of the infants had been on a home monitor for three months with five hospital readmissions for investigation of recurrent apnea. The other 6-week old infant had been on the home monitor 17 days without spells at any time (Table 2).

False alarms occurred in approximately 60% of the infants on home monitors. While one quarter of these were explained by electronic faults which could be easily appreciated and corrected, the rest caused anxiety and were a nuisance to the family. False alarms occurred more frequently in older, active infants and were often difficult to reverse. In severe cases the type of monitor was changed, often leading to a reduction in false alarming. No one type of monitor was immune from these problems.

DISCUSSION

Home monitoring of infants at risk for SIDS has been introduced as a 'stop-gap' while investigators try to discover the cause(s). To date, just as research efforts have not unravelled the etiology of SIDS (4), home monitor programs have not as yet been able to prove that SIDS deaths have been prevented.

In the program reported here two deaths of SIDS siblings occurred on well-functioning monitors (Table 2) and despite institution of cardiopulmonary re-suscitation. The reported recurrence of SIDS in a family who has lost a previous infant is 1–2% (9) and therefore 2 deaths in 126 home-monitored infants is the expected incidence in the absence of monitoring. No deaths occurred in the near-miss infants, but as approximately half the group had no spells on the home monitor (Table 2), perhaps suggesting that the initial presenting spell may not have been a potentially serious one, then the number of infants monitored may have been insufficient (10). Certainly deaths on monitors of near-miss infants have been reported by other groups (11, 12).

Over the same 9 years of home monitoring in the area the incidence of SIDS has ranged between 1.83 and 1.14 deaths per 1000 live births. Although this reported incidence is less than the death rate of 2–3 per 1000 live births reported in 1960–61 (13) there is as yet no evidence that home monitoring has led to a sustained reduction in the incidence of SIDS.

We must be careful, then, in advising parents with infants at risk for SIDS, to ensure that they appreciate that home monitoring is still experimental and that prevention of death is not guaranteed. Because all monitors will false alarm, often increasing family anxiety (14), industry should be encouraged to develop a more accurate monitoring device. As the cost of home monitoring is not inconsequential, financial considerations must be weighed against the use of an experimental device. Reporting of successes and failures in home monitor programs is necessary, just as continued research is essential to define the cause(s) of SIDS.

REFERENCES

1. Valdes-Dapena M: Sudden unexplained infant death, 1970 through 1975. An evolution in understanding. Pathol Annu 12:117–145, 1977
2. Naeye RL: Pulmonary arterial abnormalities in the sudden-infant-death syndrome. N Engl J Med 289:1167–1170, 1973
3. Naeye RL, Whalen P, Ryser M, Fisher R: Cardiac and other abnormalities in the sudden infant death syndrome. Am J Pathol 82:1–8, 1976
4. Avery ME, Frantz III ID: To breathe or not to breathe: what have we learned about apneic spells and sudden infant death? N Engl J Med 309:107–108, 1983
5. Kelly DH, Walker AM, Cahen L, Shannon DC: Periodic breathing in siblings of sudden infant death syndrome victims. Pediatrics 66:515–520, 1980
6. Hoppenbrouwers T, Hodgman JE, McGinty D, Harper RM, Sterman MB: Sudden infant death syndrome: sleep apnea and respiration in subsequent siblings. Pediatrics 66:205–214, 1980
7. Guilleminault C, Ariagno R, Korobkin R, Nagel L, Baldwin R, Coons S, Owen M: Mixed and obstructive sleep apnea and near-miss for sudden infant death syndrome. 2. Comparison of near-miss and normal control infants by age. Pediatrics 64:882–891, 1979
8. Duffty P, Bryan MH: Home apnea monitoring in near-miss sudden infant death syndrome (SIDS) and in siblings of SIDS victims. Pediatrics 70:69–74, 1982
9. Froggatt P, Lynas MA, MacKenzie G: Epidemiology of sudden unexpected death in infants ('cot deaths') in Northern Ireland. Br J Prev Soc Med 25:119–134, 1971
10. Hodgman JE, Hoppenbrouwers T, Geidel S, Hadeed A, Sterman MB, Harper R, McGinty D: Respiratory behaviour in near-miss sudden infant death syndrome. Pediatrics 69:785–792, 1982
11. Kelly DH, Shannon DC, O'Connell K: Care of infants with near-miss sudden infant death syndrome. Pediatrics 61:511–514, 1978
12. Rosen CL, Frost JD, Harrison GM: Infant apnea: polygraphic studies and follow-up monitoring. Pediatrics 71:731–736, 1983
13. Steele R, Kraus AS, Langworth JT: Sudden, unexpected death in infancy in Ontario. Part 1: methodology and findings related to the host. Can J Public Health 58:359–364, 1967
14. Nelson NM: But who shall monitor the monitor? Pediatrics 61:663–664, 1978

16. PHYSIOLOGY AS APPLIED TO PEDIATRIC ANESTHESIA

David J. Steward

David J. Steward

INTRODUCTION

The optimal anesthetic management of pediatric patients demands a broad knowledge of the physiology of infancy and childhood. Major physiological differences from the adult exist at birth, and these become less as the child grows to adolescence. The effects of surgical diseases, the operation, and general anesthesia on the normal physiolgy of the child must be considered. The respiratory and cardiovascular systems are of particular concern to the anesthetist, and there are also important metabolic considerations.

THE RESPIRATORY SYSTEM

From the time of the first breath, through infancy and childhood, the respiratory system continues to develop progressively. The physiology of the newborn and the changes during childhood will be considered, together with the changes produced by anesthetic drugs.

Control of ventilation

Control of ventilation is well developed in healthy, fullterm neonates and is dependent upon both biochemical and reflex mechanisms (1). The ventilatory response of normothermic infants to increased concentrations of inspired CO_2 is proportionally similar to that of adults. However, ventilation at any level of $PaCO_2$ is higher, reflecting the higher metabolic rate of the infant. The normal arterial CO_2 tension ($PaCO_2$) is 30–35 mmHg in the newborn, and reaches adult levels of 35–50 mmHg within a few months. The peripheral chemoreceptors are active, as demonstrated by the fact that administration of 100% oxygen produces a fall in the level of ventilation. The ventilatory response to hypoxemia in the newborn is usually an initial increase in ventilation, followed by a sustained decrease in ventilation. This decrease in ventilation following hypoxemia is even more pronounced in the preterm infant. Inhaled general anesthetic agents depress ventilation, and the $PaCO_2$ rises. The ventilatory response to hypoxemia is probably also modified by potent volatile anesthetic agents. In young adults, the increase in ventilation in response to hypoxia is inhibited 84 very low concentrations of inhaled anesthetic vapors.

Regulation of ventilation by reflexes arising in the lungs may be particularly important in neonates, especially the preterm. The Hering-Breuer stretch reflex, active in premature infants and still present at term, declines within a few months, as other mechanisms assume a major role in maintaining ventilation. Head's paradoxical reflex (a large sigh following a normal inspiration) is also active during the first few months of life: it probably plays a major role in preserving inflation of the immature lung. This reflex persists even in anesthetized babies.

Ventilation falls during general anesthesia, and the arterial carbon dioxide tension increases. This fall in the ventilation is due to a depression in the sensitivity of the central chemoreceptors to carbon dioxide, and may be partially reversed by the CNS effects of surgical stimulation. General anesthetic agents have also been demonstrated to depress ventilatory muscle function. Halothane in clinically useful concentrations severely depresses intercostal muscle activity (2). Thus, the contribution of chest wall movement is minimal during anesthesia, and ventilation becomes predominantly diaphragmatic.

Lung volumes

In the newborn, total lung capacity (TLC) is aout 160 cc and functional residual capacity (FRC) is about 80 cc. Tidal volume ($\dot{V}_T$) is 15–20 cc; one third of this is dead space ventilation. In relation to body size, these volumes are similar to adult values (3). However, in relation to the dead space of anesthetic equipment for adults, they are very small.

By contrast, alveolar ventilation ($\dot{V}_A$) is proportionally much higher in the infant than in the adult (100–150 vs 60 cc/kg/min), a difference that reflects the infant's higher metabolic rate. This large $\dot{V}_A$ results in a $\dot{V}_A$:FRC ratio of 5:1 in neonates, compared with 1.5:1 in adults. Consequently, changes in inspired gas concentrations are rapidly reflected in alveolar and arterial levels, as demonstrated by the faster equilibration of inspired and alveolar levels of inhalation anesthetic agents (4). Although the neonate's level of alveolar ventilation can meet the demands of this higher metabolic rate for O_2, any interruption of ventilation or reduction in inspired O_2 concentration is rapidly followed by arterial hypoxemia. Thus, during anesthesia, one must ensure adequate inspired O_2 concentrations and alveolar ventilation – babies go blue very quickly. The total number of alveoli present increases until approximately 10 years of age. Thus, the newborn, with fewer alveoli than the adult, has a smaller respiratory air–tissue interface. Therefore, infants have smaller reserve capability for gas exchange.

In neonates, the lung's closing volume is high (5), and normally encroaches upon $\dot{V}_T$; this contributes to the larger difference between their alveolar and arterial O_2 tensions (A/aO$_2$ difference). During anesthesia, falls in FRC at least similar to those in adults may be expected, and will further increase the A/aO$_2$ difference.

Lung mechanics

By the end of the neonatal period, an infant's total specific compliance has reached that of an adult, and similar inflating pressures are required during controlled ventilation. However, the rib cage is soft, and the chest wall compliance is very much higher, providing only a weak expansile force to maintain FRC. Intercostal muscle activity is much reduced during general anesthesia, which may account for the large falls in FRC seen during and after anesthesia.

The soft chest wall tends to move paradoxically in anesthetized infants, and this becomes marked if any obstruction to ventilation is present. As the child grows from infancy into early childhood, the rib cage becomes more rigid, and is more effective in opposing the action of the diaphragm.

The muscles of ventilation of the neonate, and especially of the preterm, are prone to fatigue. This is due to a lower proportion of fatigue-resistant, high-oxidative fibers in the diaphragm and intercostal muscles (6). The proportion of high-oxidative fibers increases progressively during the first year of life. The tendency to muscle fatigue in the preterm infant may explain the high incidence of perioperative apnea in these patients (7).

Total airway resistance is high in infants, because the airways are smaller. The normal infants's upper airway does not contribute as great a proportion as that of the adult to this total resistance. However, since neonates are obligatory nose-breathers and have narrow nasal passages, mucosal swelling or retention of nasal secretions may seriously obstruct ventilation. As the child grows, total airway resistance falls, and the proportion contributed by the upper airway increases. In children 1–4 years old, the diameter of the airway within the cricoid cartilage just below the vocal cords is crucial in determining resistance to flow; even a slight increase in this, due to edema of the lining tissue, greatly increases airway resistance. Hence, at this age patients are very susceptible to croup, due to viral infection or resultant upon the trauma of endotracheal intubation. Selection of a suitable size endotracheal tube is crucial to avoid damage to delicate subglottic tissues.

Endotracheal intubation results in an increased resistance to ventilation in most infants and children. Therefore, assisted or controlled ventilation is required during all but the shortest anesthetics.

170

Gas exchange

Efficient gas exchange in the lungs is dependent upon even matching of ventilation, and perfusion throughout the lung tissue.

Pulmonary ventilation and perfusion become quite evenly matched within the first week of life, and the PaO_2 while breathing room air increases from 75 mmHg at 24 hr to 90 mmHg at 7 days. The A/aO_2 difference is greater in infants than in adults because of anatomic shunts in the infant and the higher closing volume.

General anesthesia, muscle paralysis, and artificial ventilation all affect the distribution of ventilation within the lungs. Volatile anesthetic agents interfere with the normal control of the pulmonary blood vessels. Thus, during anesthesia, increased mismatching of ventilation and perfusion occurs, and increased levels of inspired oxygen are indicated.

THE CARDIOVASCULAR SYSTEM

In infancy, the CVS must meet the nutritional demands of a body with a high proportion of vessel-rich, metabolically active tissues (8). This is achieved by a relatively high cardiac output and large blood volume, and, in the first few weeks of life, a high hemoglobin level. As the child grows, his CVS becomes more like that in an adult. Therefore, as with the respiratory system, it is the newborn who demonstrates the greatest difference from the adult.

Cardiac output

It is difficult to measure cardiac output in neonates because of persistent fetal vascular shunts, but it is generally agreed that their cardiac output/kg body weight is 2–3 times that of adults. This is appropriate in relation to metabolic rate. Since the neonate has a high cardiac output but relatively low arterial blood pressure (BP) (9), peripheral vascular resistance must be low; this accords with the higher proportion of vessel-rich tissues. The arterial blood pressure of the infant is dependent upon maintenance of the high cardiac output, and there is less capacity for peripheral vasoconstriction than in the adult. Depression of the myocardium by potent anesthetic agents rapidly decreases cardiac output and, consequently, arterial BP. Therefore, care must be taken to avoid giving excessive amounts of these agents, particularly during controlled ventilation. Excessive preoperative fluid restriction may also increase the likelihood of hypotension in response to general anesthetic agents.

Blood volume

Average blood volume in neonates is approximately 84 ml/kg body weight; this falls to 75 ml/kg body weight at 6 weeks, 72 ml/kg body weight at 2 years, and 60–70 ml/kg body weight at puberty. A decrease in blood volume such as might occur during surgical bleeding is accompanied in the infant by a progressive fall in systolic arterial BP; pressure is restored when the blood volume is replaced (10, 11). This suggests that the neonate's capacity to adjust his vascular volume to the available blood volume is not fully developed. The baroreceptor response of infants to changes in blood pressure is absent during anesthesia (12). These findings agree with the experience of pediatric anesthesiologists that changes in systolic arterial BP parallel changes in the circulating blood volume. In infants, a fall in blood volume is closely followed by a fall in cardiac output and in systolic BP. Thus, if O_2 transport is to be maintained, blood losses must be replaced promptly. The systolic BP is the most accurate clinical guide to adequate blood replacement in small infants.

Response of the cardiovascular system to hypoxemia

Hypoxia is an ever-present danger during anesthesia and must be recognized rapidly. In contrast to adults, in whom the initial response to hypoxia usually is tachycardia, babies demonstrate bradycardia as the first sign (13). Thus, during anesthesia hypoxemia must be suspected immediately if bradycardia occurs and the O_2 level in the inspired gases and pulmonary ventilation must be checked immediately.

Hypoxemia in the fetus and newborn is followed by systemic vasoconstriction, in contrast to the adult in whom vasodilation occurs. Thus, hypoxemia has a disastrous effect on oxygen transport in the newborn.

Hemoglobin

At birth, 70% of the blood's hemoglobin content is of the fetal type (Hb F); then, during the first few months, the Hb F decreases as it is replaced with adult-type hemoglobin (Hb A). Total Hb = 16–18 g/dl at birth, decreasing to 10–11 g/dl by 3 months and increasing to 14–15 g/dl by puberty.

If an otherwise healthy child is found to be anemic when examined pre-operatively, elective surgery should be deferred until this has been investigated and treated. Any significant degree of anemia reduces the blood's O_2-carrying capacity and reduces the margin of safety in the event that O_2 delivery to the lungs is interrupted – hence, the greater incidence of cardiac arrest during anesthesia in infants and children who are anemic (14).

The minimum acceptable level of the hemoglobin for elective surgery in older infants and children is generally considered to be 10 g/dl. Young infants, and especially those with cardiorespiratory disease, require higher levels of at least 14 g/dl.

THERMOREGULATION

Small babies lose body heat rapidly if placed in a cool environment. This is chiefly because of their small total body mass and disproportionately large body surface area; absence of a heat-insulating layer of fat and less effective control of superficial blood vessels are contributing factors. Thus, even if a neonate's thermoregulatory control mechanisms are well developed, he will suffer wide variations in body temperature if endogenous heat production cannot balance excessive heat loss. Anesthesia, especially with agents such as halothane that cause peripheral vasodilation, further increases heat loss (15).

When heat loss occurs, the body responds by increasing heat production to attempt to prevent a fall in body core temperature. Adults and children over a few months of age respond with increased skeletomuscular activity (shivering): this reaction can be blocked by muscle relaxants. Neonates cannot shiver effectively; their response to the need to produce more heat consists of a general increase in metabolism and markedly accelerated metabolic activity in certain tissues, particularly the brown adipose tissue. The latter tissue, located chiefly in the interscapular region, has a very rich blood supply; when metabolically active, its O_2 consumption can approach that of even cardiac muscle.

In neonates, control of this heat-producing mechanism is mediated by the sympathetic nervous system and is dependent upon skin thermoreceptors sensitive to environmental changes. Thus, the newborn's skin temperature powerfully influences his metaolic rate. His O_2 uptake is minimal when his skin temperature is maintained at 36–37° C.

Measurements of O_2 uptake in anesthetized babies show no difference from the awake state, and mild degrees of hypothermia may be associated with a greatly increased uptake (16). Neuromuscular blocking agents probably do not decrease O_2 uptake in hypothermic neonates as they do in hypothermic adult patients.

RENAL FUNCTION AND FLUID BALANCE

Renal function in babies over 1 month of age is physiologically similar to that in adults. Such infants can excrete drugs via the kidneys, produce large volumes of dilute urine in response to a fluid load, conserve sodium when necessary, and concentrate urine when they are fluid depleted. Younger infants, especially neonates, respond to these challenges less effectively (17).

Glomerular filtration

The glomerular filtration rate (GFR) is low in the immediate newborn period, and increases over the first weeks of life. GFR is lower in preterm infants, and does not increase as rapidly as in the term infant. The low GFR limits the ability of the young infant to excrete a fluid load rapidly, or to excrete excess electrolytes. Therefore, fluid administration during anesthesia must be carefully controlled. GFR is further reduced in neonatal illnesses, especially when congestive heart failure, sepsis, and/or hypoxemia are present.

Tubular function

Tubular function is limited in the neonate, and progressively improves over the first weeks of life. Therefore, conservation or excretion of electrolytes and other substances is limited. Sodium reabsorption in the tubule is limited and thus, sodium may be lost during excretion of a hypotonic fluid load. Glucose reabsorption is also limited, and this results in a low renal threshold for glucose. Excessive glucose administration to small infants may result in glycosuria, and the resultant osmotic diuresis can lead to severe dehydration. The renal tubular capacity to conserve bicarbonate and to compensate for acid–base disturbances is limited in the neonate.

Fluid balance

Fluid distribution within the body compartments is different in infants, in whom the extracellular fluid compartment is much larger. Therefore, they may have to be given relatively larger doses of drugs that are distributed within this space.

Fluid turnover is slow until about 24 hr after birth, at which time it rapidly increases to a rate exceeding that in older children and adults. Consequently, any limitation of fluid intake in infants and young children, however healthy they may be, rapidly results in dehydration.

Insensible fluid loss in small infants is increased when overhead radiant heaters or 'bili' lights are in use.

Fluid management

In small infants, fluid administration must be very carefully controlled. Infusion pumps and low volume infusion sets should be employed. Small syringes (tuberculin) should be used to accurately measure small doses of drugs.

The most important considerations in planning the perioperative fluid manage-

174

ment of healthy children are to minimize the preoperative fasting period (18, 19), and to use techniques least likely to delay the return of normal appetite and fluid intake. Parents of outpatients must be given written instructions about fluid and food intake preoperatively and about the importance of adequate fluids postoperatively. The preoperative fasting orders for outpatients at The Hospital for Sick Children are as follows:

1. Infants under 2 years of age should be given clear fluids until 4 hr before surgery. Other feedings must be discontinued at east 6 hr preoperatively.
2. Children over 2 years of age must have no food on the day of operation, but may be offered clear fluids up to 4 hr preoperatively.

With this regime, the child arrives for surgery in a good state of hydration, although he may have a mild metabolic acidosis. Preoperative fluid administration must take into account the type and probable duration of surgery and the anticipated time until resumption of oral intake. Most children undergoing minor surgery as outpatients really do not require infusion of fluids. If the procedure is lengthy, an infusion should be given at a rate calculated to make up the preoperative fluid deficit, provide maintenance and replace losses during surgery.

Maintenance fluids (usually 5% dextrose with 0.2 N saline) are given according to the following scale: under 1 month of age, 3 ml/kg/hr; 1 month–1 year, 6 ml/kg/hr; 1–2 years, 4 ml/kg/hr; and over 2 year, 3 ml/kg/hr. The infusion rate during the first hour of surgery is adjusted to include replacement of the deficit from the fasting period. Thus, for a child over 2 years of age who has had no fluids for 4 hr, 15 ml/kg/hr would be given during the first hour; subsequently, fluid administration would be reduced to maintenance levels.

Fluids for infants and small children must be warmed, and the intravenous set must permit the accurate administration of small volumes and not be subject to sudden accidental infusion of large amounts. No more than 250 ml should be in place for any patient weighing less than 30 kg, and a controlled infusion set (e.g. Pedatrol of Buretrol) must be used to administer fluids in suitable aliquots. An infusion pump should be used for infants.

REFERENCES

1. Bryan AC, Bryan MH: Control of respiration in the newborn. Clin Perinatol 5:270–281, 1978
2. Tusiewicz J, Bryan AC, Froese AB: Contributions of changing R.B. cage–diaphragm interactions to the ventilatory depression of halothane anesthesia. Anesthesiology 47:327–337, 1977
3. Nelson NM: Neonatal pulmonary function. Ped Clin North Am 13:769–799, 1966
4. Steward DJ, Creighton RE: The uptake and excretion of nitrous oxide in the newborn. Can Anaesth Soc J 25:215, 1978
5. Mansell A, Bryan AC, Levison H: Airway closure in children. J Appl Physiol 33:711–714, 1972
6. Muller N, Gulston G, Cade D et al: Diaphragmatic muscle fatigue in the newborn. J Appl Physiol 44:909–913, 1978
7. Steward DJ: Preterm infants are more prone to complications following minor surgery than are term infants. Anesthesiology 56:304–306, 1982

8. Friis Hansen B: Body composition during growth. Pediatrics 47:264–274, 1971

9. Versmold HT, Kitterman JA, Phibbs RH, Gregory GA, Tooley WH: Aortic blood pressure during the first 12 hours of life in infants with birth weight 610 to 4220 grams. Pediatrics 67:607–613, 1981

10. Wallgren G, Barr M, Rudhe U: Hemodynamic studies of induced acute hypo- and hypervolemia in the newborn infant. Acta Paed Scan 53:1, 1964

11. Wallgren G, Hansen JS, Lind J: Quantitative studies of the human neonatal circulation III. Observations on the newborn infant's central circulatory responses to moderate hypovolemia. Acta Paed Scand (Suppl) 179:43, 1967

12. Gregory GA: The baroresponses of preterm infants during halothane anaesthesia. Can Anaesth Soc J 29:105–107, 1982

13. James LS, Rowe RD: The pattern of response of pulmonary and systemic arterial pressures in newborn and older infants to short periods of hypoxia. J Pediat 51:5, 1957

14. Salem MR, Bennett EJ, Schweiss J, Baraka A, Dalal FY, Collins VJ: Cardiac arrest related to anesthesia contributing factors in infants and children. JAMA 233:238–241, 1975

15. Engelman DR, Lockhart CH: Comparisons between temperature effects of ketamine and halothane anesthesia in children. Anesth Analg (Cleve) 51:98, 1972

16. Ryan JF, Wilson RS, Goudsouzian NG, Jasinska MT: Oxygen consumption as a measure of thermoregulation in children. Abstract of the Annual Meeting, American Society of Anesthesiologists, San Francisco, pp 273–274, 1973

17. Guignard JP: Renal function in the newborn infant. Ped Clin North Amer 29:777, 1982

18. Thomas DKM: Hypoglycaemia in children before operaton: its incidence and prevention. Br J Anaesth 46:66, 1974

19. Watson BG: Blood glucose levels in children during surgery. Br J Anaesth 44:712, 1972

17. STRUCTURAL DEVELOPMENT OF THE PULMONARY CIRCULATION AND MYOCARDIUM

MARLENE RABINOVITCH

INTRODUCTION

> [The triangle] is nature's basic structure
> ... R. Buckminster Fuller

In the infant and young child, the cardiovascular response to stress is determined by the state of structural development of a triad of elements – the pulmonary vascular bed, the systemic vascular bed and the myocardium. A chronic hemo-dynamic change will in turn disturb the normal process of vascular and myocar-dial growth and remodelling. Therefore, the ability to advantageously manipul-ate the developing circulatory system both functionally and structurally is the goal of current patient management and future research.

THE PULMONARY VASCULAR BED

Normal development

Applying a technique of arterial injection to postmortem lung specimens (1) of fetus, newborn and child, the normal pattern of growth and remodelling of the pulmonary vascular bed was established by Elliott and Reid (2), Davies and Reid (3), and Hislop and Reid (4). The pulmonary arteries were injected at a control-led constant temperature with a radiopaque barium-gelantin mixture and the lung was subsequently inflated with formalin through the bronchial tree. By distend-ing the arteries before fixation, measurements of their external diameter at a given airway level and their wall thickness at a given external diameter were found to be consistent and precise.

It was observed that preacinar arteries follow the development of the airways and intraacinar arteries, the terminal respiratory units and alveoli. Hence the preacinar arteries are all present by the sixteenth week of gestation whereas the intraacinar arteries continue to multiply after birth until the age of eight years whereafter they increase primarily in size. Indeed, on postmortem arteriograms, the size of the preacinar arteries is seen to increase with age against an increasingly dense 'background haze' of contrast material representing the addition of intraacinar arteries not present at birth (Figure 1).

The preacinar arteries are muscular at birth but by landmarking the intraacinar arteries according to their accompanying airway, it is observed that the completely muscular coat at the level of the terminal bronchioles becomes a partially muscular coat or 'spiral of muscle' at the level of the respiratory bronchioles which then becomes nonmuscular at the level of the alveolar ducts and walls.

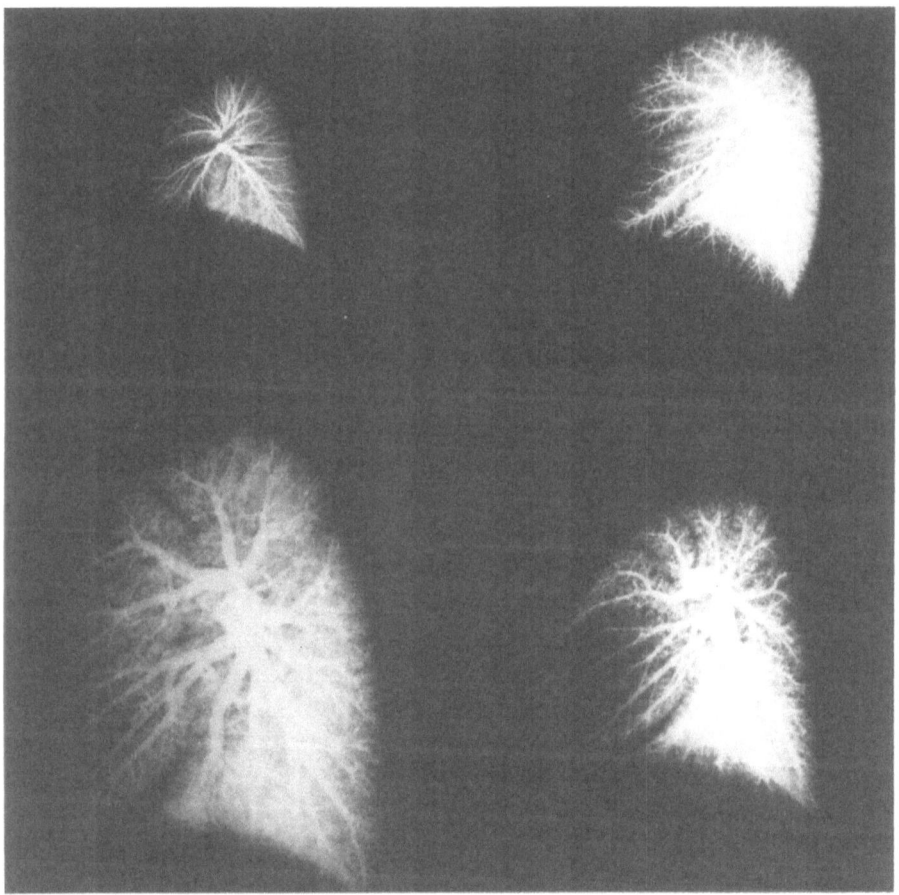

Figure 1. Postmortem arteriograms from a newborn (upper left), a three-month old (upper right), a 1-year old (lower right), and a 10-year old child (lower left). The preacinar distribution is complete in the newborn but with increasing age, the background becomes filled in by a dense haze due to the addition and growth of many small intraacinar arteries. (Reproduced with permission Moss' Heart Disease in Infants, Children and Adolescents, ed: FH Adams, Emmanovilides GC, 1983. Williams and Williams, Baltimore.)

With increasing age, however, muscle is seen to 'extend' into arteries located more peripherally within the acinus (Figure 2). Thus, in the two-year old child, fully muscular arteries are apparent, accompanying the respiratory bronchioli, and in the eight-year old child they are present alongside the alveolar ducts; in the adult they are occasionally seen at alveolar wall level. The stimulus for the appearance of new muscle in peripheral arteries is unknown but it seems that perhaps vessels must grow to a certain size before they acquire a muscular coat, i.e. the terminal bronchiolus artery of the newborn is the same diameter as the alveolar wall artery in the adult. In ultrastructural studies by Meyrick and Reid (5) the appearance of new muscle has been shown to be due to the differentiation of precursor cells, the pericyte in the normally nonmuscular region of the artery and the intermediate cell in the partially muscular region to mature smooth muscle.

The normally muscular arteries are most thick-walled in the fetus and newborn. With the drop in pulmonary vascular resistance at birth, vessels dilate, and

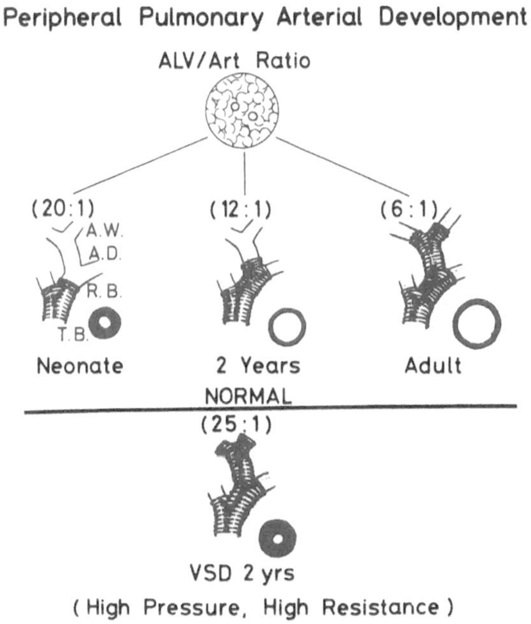

Figure 2. Schema showing (in upper panel) normal peripheral pulmonary arterial development: extension of muscle into peripheral arteries, percent wall thickness, and artery number (alveolar arterial ratio) as they relate to age. Lower panel shows abnormalities in all three features in a 2-year old child with a hypertensive VSD (ventricular septal defect).
T.B. = artery accompanying terminal bronchiolus.
R.B. = artery accompanying respiratory bronchiolus.
A.D. = artery accompanying alveolar duct.
A.W. = artery accompanying alveolar wall.
(Reproduced with permission (68).)

there is also some regression of the medial musculature. Thus, wall thickness, when expressed as a percent of external diameter, has thinned to the adult level in arteries <250 μM within the first few days of life and in arteries of all sizes within the first four months. This is in keeping with hemodynamic studies which show the greatest drop in pulmonary artery pressure within the first few days of life – but continuing to about six weeks of life when adult levels are achieved (6).

Arteries keep pace with multiplication of alveoli but 'steal' a little ahead so that whereas in the newborn there is one artery for every 20 alveoli, the two-year old has one artery for every 12 and the adult, one artery for every six alveoli.

In any patient, the features of growth and muscularity of the arteries can be quantified and compared to normal values for age. Because of the uniform distribution of these structural features, even a small biopsy section of 1 cm^2 is representative of the lung as a whole (7). This method of morphometric analysis

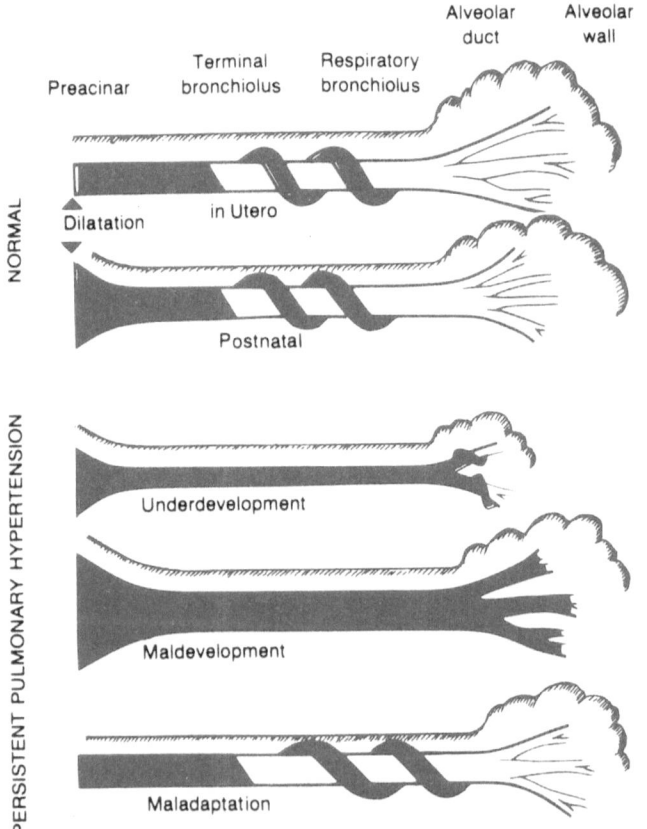

Figure 3. Schema showing normal arterial dilatation during transition from fetal to neonatal circulation. When the lung is underdeveloped the vascular bed is hypoplastic and abnormally muscular; when it is maldeveloped the arteries are abnormally muscular, and when it is maladapted, it has not dilated appropriately at birth. (Adapted from L Reid.)

of the features of growth and remodelling of the pulmonary vascular bed has been applied to the lungs of infants and children with a variety of disease states. In almost all cases, the severity of structural abnormalities could be judged from a small section of injected lung tissue.

Persistent pulmonary hypertension of the newborn

Persistent pulmonary hypertension of the newborn which has been loosely called 'persistence of the fetal circulaltion' because of associated atrial and/or ductal right to left shunting, may result from one of three causes: (i) underdevelopment of the lung and pulmonary vascular bed; (ii) maldevelopment of the pulmonary vascular bed; or (iii) maladaptation of the pulmonary vascular bed (Figure 3). The first two causes probably result from intrauterine insults sustained at dif-

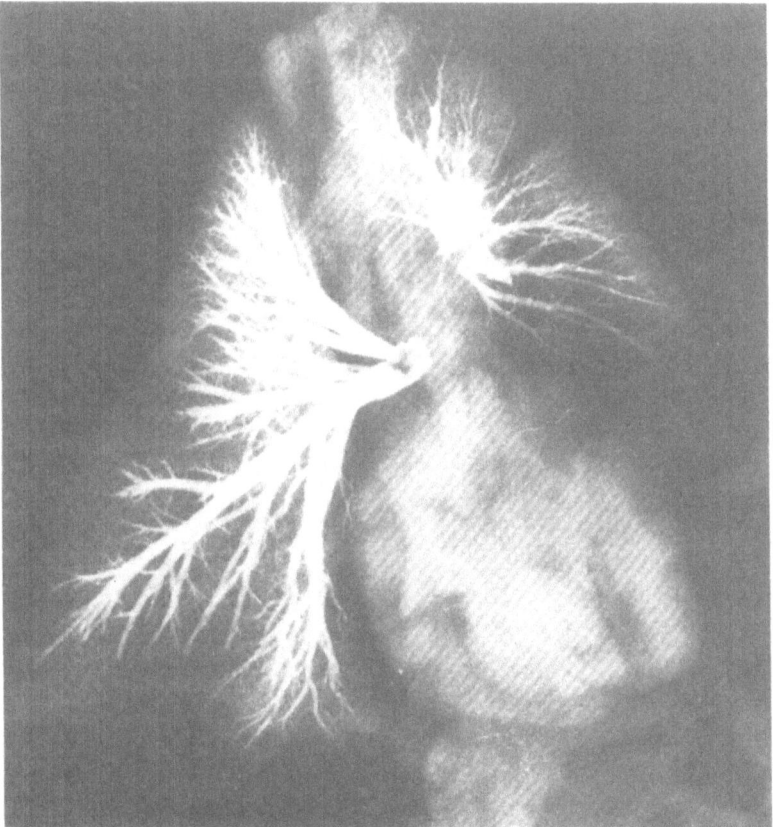

Figure 4. Postmortem arteriogram in an infant with congenital diaphragmatic hernia; right lung is small, the left lung much smaller, arteries in both lungs are reduced in size and number. (Reproduced with permission (8).)

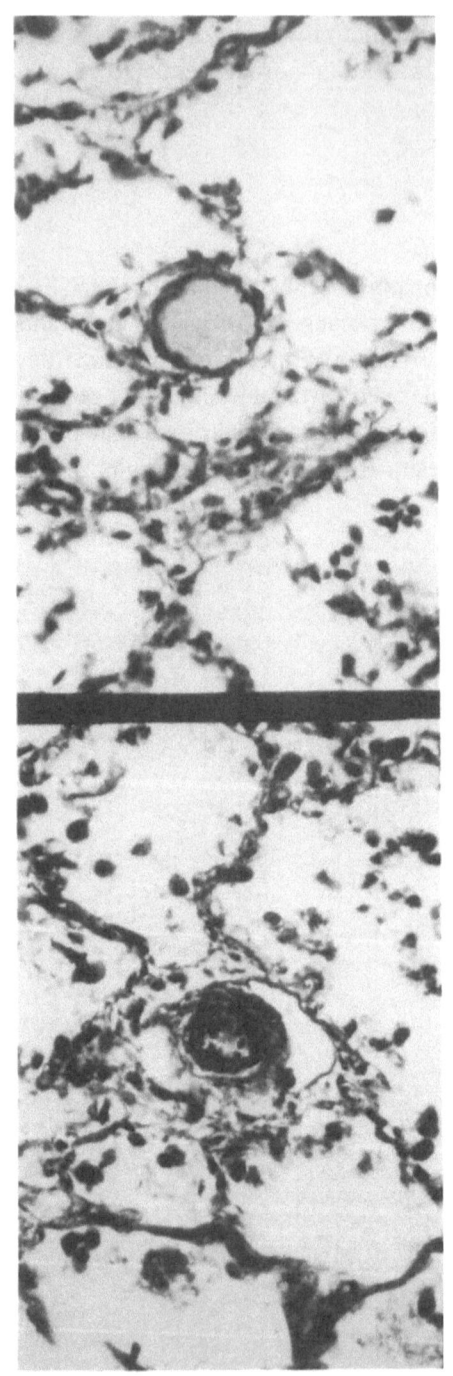

Figure 5. Photomicrographs of alveolar wall arteries injected at postmortem with a barium-gelatin suspension. LHS shows a normal nonmuscular artery from a three-day old infant who had a normal heart and lungs. RHS shows an abnormally muscularized artery from an infant with persistent pulmonary hypertension. Elastic Van Gieson ×250. (Reproduced with permission (24).)

ferent critical periods during gestation whereas the third is likely the response to a perinatal insult.

Underdevelopment of the pulmonary vascular bed
Congenital diaphragmatic hernia is an example of underdevelopment of the pulmonary vascular bed (8, 9). Peripheral arteries are reduced in proportion to the diminished lung volume and the decrease in total alveolar number (Figure 4). Both this feature, causing resistance to pulmonary blood flow, and the severe hypoxia and hypercarbia, resulting from decreased gas exchange surface area, account for the severe pulmonary hypertension and right to left shunting from birth. Depending upon the severity of the structural abnormalities, the hemo-dynamic derangement will either reverse after surgical correction of the diaphrag-matic defect, or after the concomitant institution of therapy with vasodilators such as tolazoline (10), or with the extracorporeal membrane oxygenator (11), or will be irreversible. Other conditions associated with pulmonary hypertension as a result of lung and vascular hypoplasia include renal agenesis and dysplasia (12), rhesus isoimmunization (13), prematurity (14), asphyxiating thoracic dystrophy, and absence of the phrenic nerve (15).

Maladaptation of the pulmonary vascular bed
Infants with perinatal stress from a variety of causes, e.g. hemorrhage, hypo-glycemia, aspiration or hypoxia, may fail to demonstrate the normal drop in pulmonary vascular resistance at birth (16, 17, 18). The normally muscular ar-teries, in particular those $<250\,\mu M$, fail to dilate, and left ventricular dysfunction likely contributes as well (19). Of all types of persistent pulmonary hypertension, this should be the most amenable to improvement following correction of the primary disorder, using as adjunctive therapy hyperventilation (20) or vasodila-tors (21, 22).

Maldevelopment of the pulmonary vascular bed
There is a group of newborn infants who manifest persistent pulmonary hyperten-sion either in association with meconium aspiration or for no apparent reason, and who prove refractory to vasodilator therapy and succumb usually within the first few days of life. Haworth and Reid (23) and Murphy et al. (18, 24) examined lungs at postmortem in these infants and observed normal growth of the pulmo-nary vascular bed but a striking appearance of muscle in arteries small and peripheral in location and normally nonmuscular. The muscle cells were sur-rounded by darkly staining elastic laminae suggesting that they had formed several weeks prior to death and therefore in utero (Figure 5). McKenzie and Haworth reported a fatal case of persistent pulmonary hypertension of the newborn in which, in addition to abnormal muscularization, arterial size and number were decreased, suggesting loss of arteries and impaired growth (25). In addition, the lumen of the remaining peripheral arteries was partially or com-

pletely occluded by swollen endothelial cells (25). These structurally deranged cells might be impaired in their ability to handle or produce vasoactive substances (26, 27). A disproportionate increase in vasoconstrictors could theoretically result, further contributing to the pulmonary hypertension. Levin et al. have observed platelet fibrin microthrombi in the small vessels of some infants with persistent pulmonary hypertension suggesting a perinatal coagulopathy (28). Coagulation abnormalities in the sick newborn have been described by Andrew et al. (29).

In clinical and experimental studies (30–34), a relationship has been suggested between maternal ingestion of prostaglandin synthetase inhibitors, either aspirin or indomethacin, and persistent pulmonary hypertension of the newborn associated with structural changes in the pulmonary vascular bed. Since it has been difficult to consistently demonstrate cause and effect, the association probably explains the syndrome in a few susceptible neonates. Recent studies, in general, have contributed greatly to our understanding of the vascular effects of products of the lipoxygenase and cyclooxygenase pathways of arachidonic acid metabolism (34–40). In the fetal and neonatal animals, PGE_1, 6-keto PGE_1 and PGI_2 are potent vasodilators with both pulmonary and systemic effects, whereas $PGF_2\alpha$ is a vasocontrictor; PGD_2 behaves differently depending on the age of the animal: in the fetal goat it is a vasodilator but in the newborn animal (38) a vasoconstrictor. Thus induction of certain pathways at birth may be responsible for pulmonary vasodilatation and lack of induction for vasoconstriction. The leukotrienes, potent pulmonary vasoconstrictors (40), are increased in infants with respiratory distress (41). Indomethacin given to a newborn lamb retards but does not prevent the normal fall in pulmonary vascular resistance at birth (42), but this is perhaps because its effects are not directed against a specific dilator prostaglandin.

Functional adaptation of newborn pulmonary vascular bed to acute stress

Structural determinants
Studies by James and Rowe (43) first showed that the human newborn pulmonary vascular bed was more reactive than the adult to acute hypoxia. This was attributed to the fact that the arteries at the site of pulmonary vascular resistance (44) were more muscular in the newborn than the adult, and there is experimental data to support the association between the amount of vascular smooth muscle and the degree of reactivity of the pulmonary vascular bed (45). Factors separate from hypoxia which appear to trigger severe pulmonary vasoconstriction in the newborn include acidosis (46–49), polycythemia and/or hypervolemia (50, 51). The latter may not only be a feature of the muscular pulmonary vascular bed but may also represent the limited ability of the newborn lung to recruit vessels (34, 52–55) suggesting that it might be particularly compromised if challenged with a volume load. There is also experimental evidence to suggest that the pulmonary

lymphatic system functions differently in the newborn (56); more lymph is produced for a given circulatory load, and this may additionally diminish the capacity of the circulation.

Neurohumoral determinants
Neither sympathetic nor parasympathetic neural supply seem to play a major role in the hemodynamic response of the newborn pulmonary vascular bed to stress (57–60). Although in canine pulmonary arteries postnatal development of histamine receptors has been shown, there is little evidence that this significantly affects pulmonary vascular responsivity (61). The metabolic function of the pulmonary vascular endothelium of the newborn, however, may be particularly vulnerable and this may result in inappropriate handling of vasoactive substances (62, 63).

Structural adaptation of the fetal and newborn pulmonary vascular bed to the chronic hemodynamic stress of a congenital heart defect

In utero
Despite the relatively small proportion of pulmonary blood flow in utero, the altered hemodynamics resulting from a congenital heart defect will affect the structure and growth of the pulmonary arteries. For example, in patients with an absent pulmonary valve, the wide pulmonary artery pulse pressure in utero is quite likely the cause of the abnormal proliferation of segmental branches which we have observed (64). These vessels are like tentacles which entwine and compress the bronchi all along their route from hilum to periphery (Figure 6). They are, in addition, to the large central pulmonary arteries which compress the main stem bronchi, a major cause of the severe (often fatal) respiratory difficulty these infants experience in the postnatal period.

In patients with pulmonary atresia and intact ventricular septum, the pulmonary arteries which develop in utero under a condition of low flow, are small, few in number and relatively nonmuscular (65). Thus, hyperreactivity may not be a problem, but inability to dilate or recruit peripheral arteries in response to a sudden increase in flow (e.g. a surgically created systemic to pulmonary artery shunt) may be responsible for the high mortality in this group of patients. In infants who have elevated pulmonary venous pressure in utero as a result of left-sided obstruction, e.g. hypoplastic left heart or obstructed total anomalous pulmonary venous drainage, a large number of excessively muscular peripheral pulmonary arteries is apparent (66, 67) (Figure 7). In patients with total anomalous pulmonary venous drainage the hyperreactivity of the pulmonary circulation in the postoperative period often causes a sustained elevation in pulmonary artery pressure which may seriously compromise cardiac output.

186

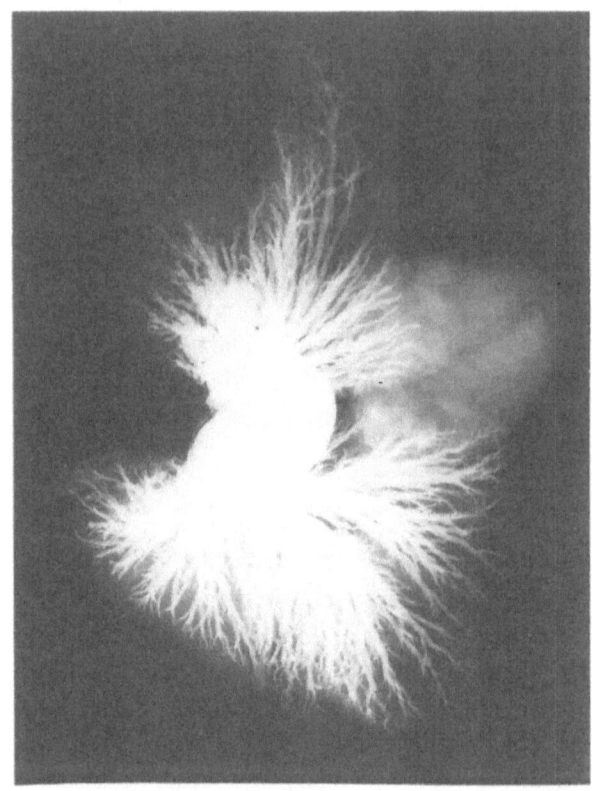

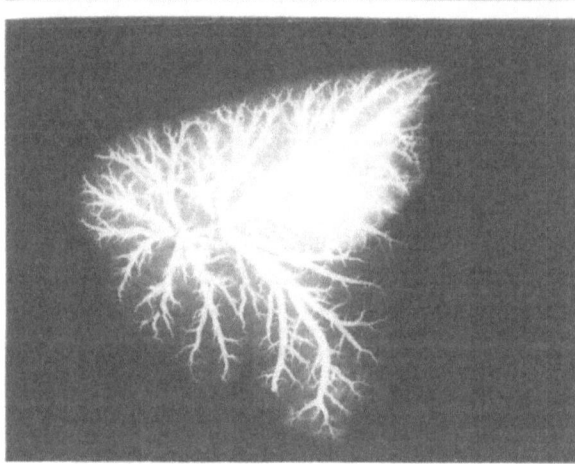

Figure 6. Postmortem arteriogram on LHS from a 10-day old infant with normal heart and lungs, and on RHS from a 10-day old infant with an absent pulmonary valve. There is a profusion of segmental pulmonary arteries. (Reproduced with permission (64).)

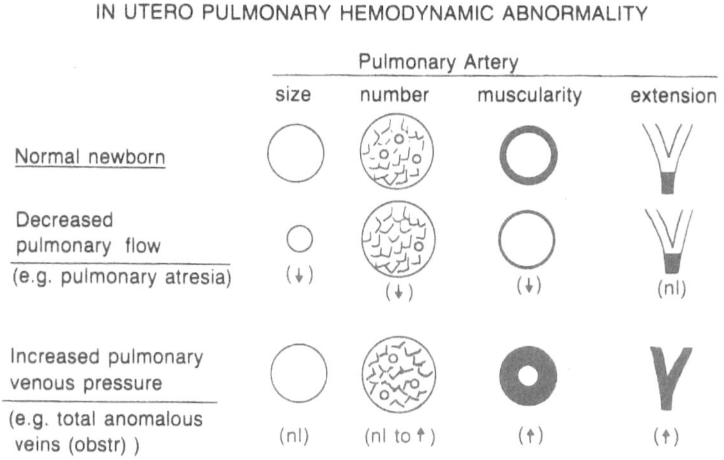

IN UTERO PULMONARY HEMODYNAMIC ABNORMALITY

Figure 7. Schema showing abnormal 'in utero' pulmonary arterial development associated with congenital heart defects. Decreased pulmonary flow is associated with hypoplasia of the peripheral pulmonary arteries, increased pulmonary venous pressure with excessive muscularity.

Postnatal

Because of the high pulmonary vascular resistance in utero congenital heart defects cause high pulmonary blood flow only after birth and therefore affect the features of *postnatal* growth and remodelling of the pulmonary vascular bed (68). The severity of the structural abnormalities can be quantitated and correlated with the degree of altered pulmonary hemodynamics. They can be graded accordingly.

Grade A: There is 'precocious' extension of muscle into arteries small and peripheral in location and normally nonmuscular for the age of the child as the sole structural abnormality, or there may be, in addition, some slight failure of the fetal musculature to dilate, but the percent medial wall thickness is ≤15% of the vessel's external diameter, normal being ≤10%. Patients with grade A changes may have increased pulmonary blood flow and pulse pressure but mean pulmonary artery pressure is generally normal.

Grade B: There are features as in A but a more severe increase in medial hypertrophy, subdivided into B (mild) when percent wall thickness is >15 <20%) and B (severe) when it is ≥20%. Patients with grade B changes have increased pulmonary blood flow; elevated mean pulmonary artery pressure is common with B (mild) and invariable with B (severe).

Grade C: In addition to the features of B (severe), there is a reduced concentration of small peripheral arteries generally accompanied by a decrease in their size as well. This feature is subdivided into C (mild) when more than half the number of peripheral arteries is present, and C (severe) when less than half is present. Patients with grade C changes tend to have elevated pulmonary vascular resistance, i.e. a disproportionate elevation in pressure relative to the increase in pulmonary blood flow.

Of the morphometric structural features, grade B (severe) is probably equivalent to Heath and Edwards' grade I (69) as medial hypertrophy can be appreciated qualitatively: grade C, the reduced arterial concentration is a new feature which can be seen alone but is common when there is mild concentric intimal hyperplasia (Heath and Edwards' grade II) and invariable when the lumen is occluded (grade III).

Patients with only grade B (severe) – Heath and Edwards' grade I vascular changes frequently demonstrate heightened reactivity of the pulmonary vascular bed in the early postoperative period following repair of a congenital heart defect (Figure 8). That is, pulmonary pressure may be as high or higher than that

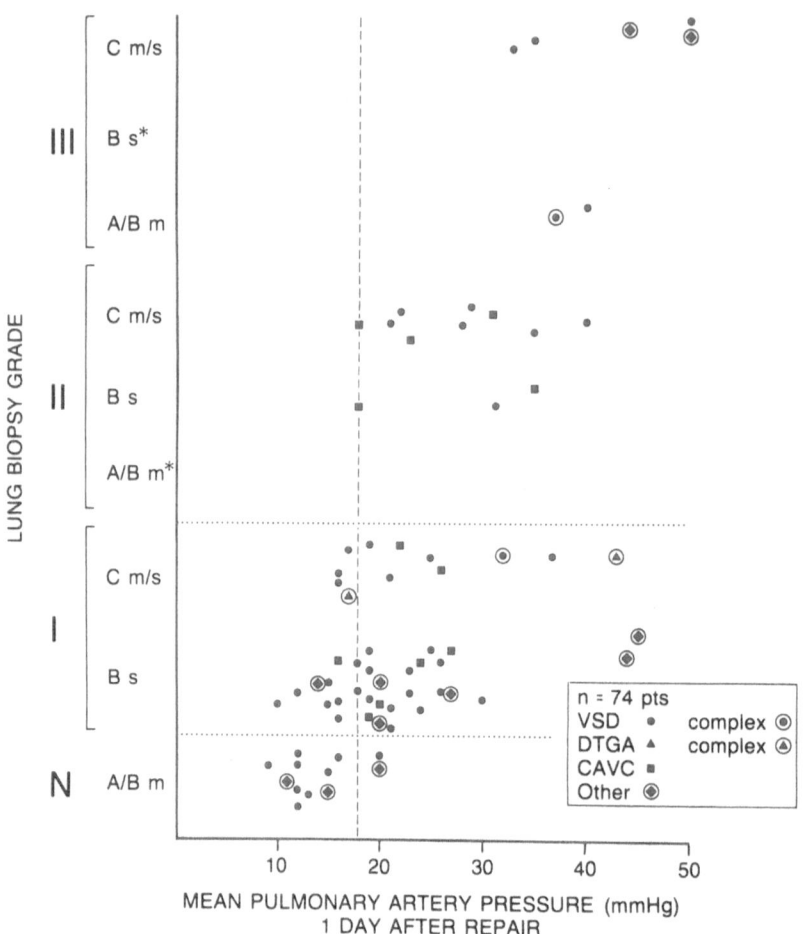

Figure 8. Graph of mean pulmonary artery pressure values the day after surgical repair of a congenital heart defect related to lung biopsy grade. Even patients with grade B changes may have severe postoperative pulmonary hypertension. (Reproduced with permission (70).)

observed preoperatively. The postoperative stimuli which may generate this pulmonary hypertension include hypoxia, acidosis (71) or perhaps release of thromboxane from platelets damaged after cardiopulmonary bypass (72).

We have recently observed an increase in factor VIII:R Ag (von Willebrand factor) in the plasma of children with congenital heart defects and pulmonary hypertension (73). The latter is produced by pulmonary vascular endothelium and an increase in its concentration may be observed in lung tissue sections that have been stained for factor VIII with immunoperoxidase. This suggests that perhaps deposition of platelet fibrin microthrombi is facilitated in the hypertensive vascular bed. Moreover, the appearance of pulmonary vascular endothelium both on scanning and transmission electron microscopy is altered in patients with pulmonary hypertension (74). The endothelial surface is uneven and deeply ridged suggesting an environment in which platelets or other leukocytes may become traumatized and perhaps release vasoconstrictor substances such as thromboxane A_2 or as leukotrienes (75) (Figure 9). The individual endothelial cells show an altered distribution of intracytoplasmic components. There are more filaments and the endoplasmic reticulum is dilated. The former may imply that the endothelial cells themselves are developing an enhanced contractile mechanism (Figure 10).

In patients with medial hypertrophy on the biopsy tissue, the reactive pulmonary hypertension encountered in the postoperative period is usually successfully managed with vasodilator therapy. One year after repair, these patients have normal levels of pulmonary artery pressure and an appropriate response to hypoxia suggesting a 'fully recovered' pulmonary vascular bed. Patients with a reduced arterial concentration and particularly those with intimal hyperplasia will invariably demonstrate heightened pulmonary vascular reactivity (70) in the early postoperative period. Only those operated within the first nine months of life however will consistently have normal pulmonary artery pressure and resistance one year after repair. This is likely because those operated upon beyond this age are probably less able to grow 'new' normal arteries (Figure 11).

Structural adaptation of the newborn pulmonary vascular bed to hypoxia – hyperoxia

Both chronic hypoxia resulting from pulmonary disease in the newborn and infant and chronic hyperoxia as a consequence of high oxygen therapy will alter the course of normal growth and structural development of pulmonary arteries (76). In experimental studies in the infant rat, chronic hypoxia results in the presence of muscle in normally nonmuscular peripheral arteries and in medial hypertrophy of normally muscular arteries. Arterial concentration is also reduced (55, 77). These changes are more severe than in the animal exposed to hypoxia from adulthood, and are less likely to reverse (Figure 12).

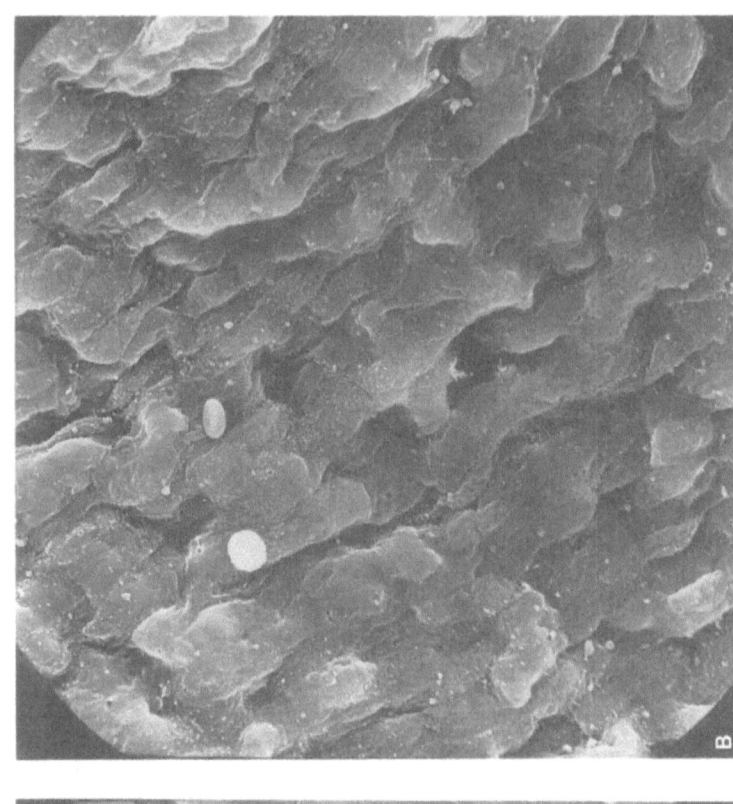

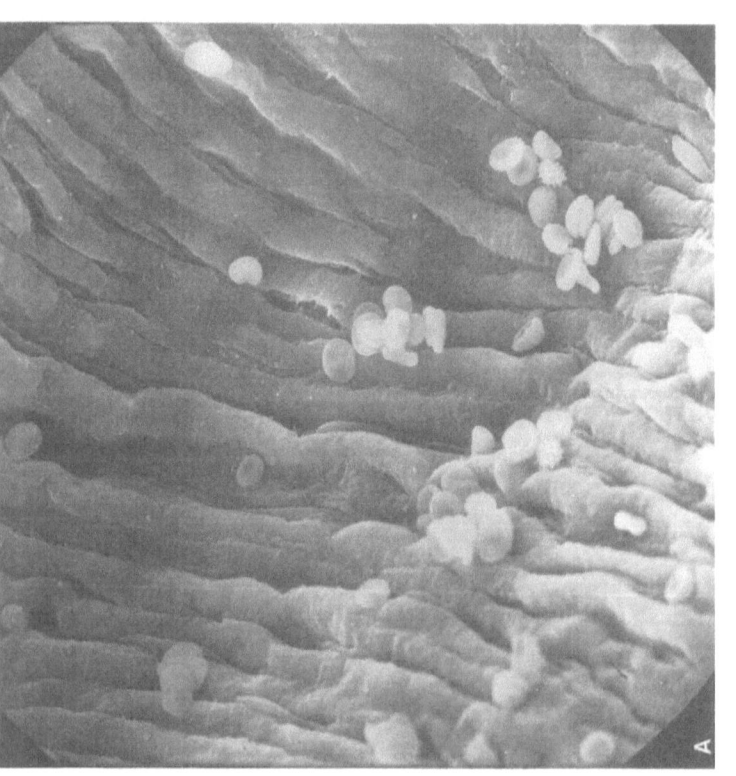

Figure 9. Scanning electron photomicrographs of pulmonary artery endothelial surfaces. A. Normal pulmonary artery shows 'corduroy pattern', neat closely aligned ridges; B. Hypertensive pulmonary artery shows 'cable' pattern, deep knotted ridges, and numerous microvilli (mV); ×810.

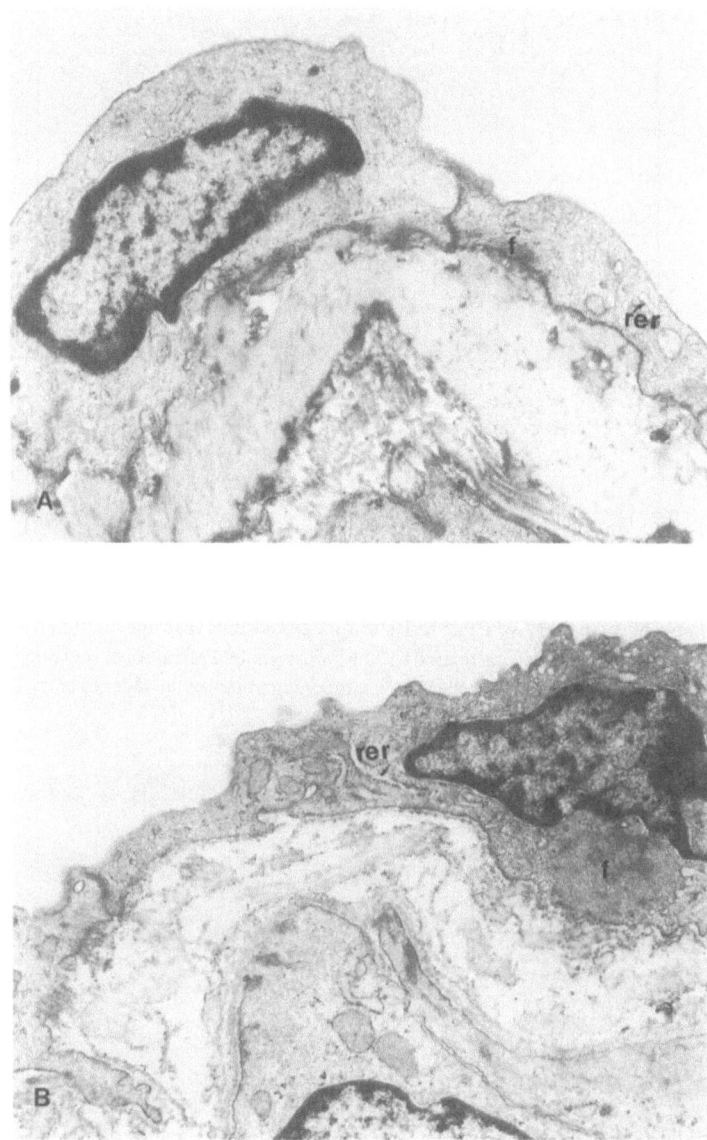

Figure 10. Transmission electron photomicrographs of pulmonary artery endothelial cells. A. Cell from normal artery shows delicate filaments in cytoplasm; B. cell from hypertensive artery shows bundles of filaments (f) and a dilated rough endoplasmic reticulum (rer); ×17 500.

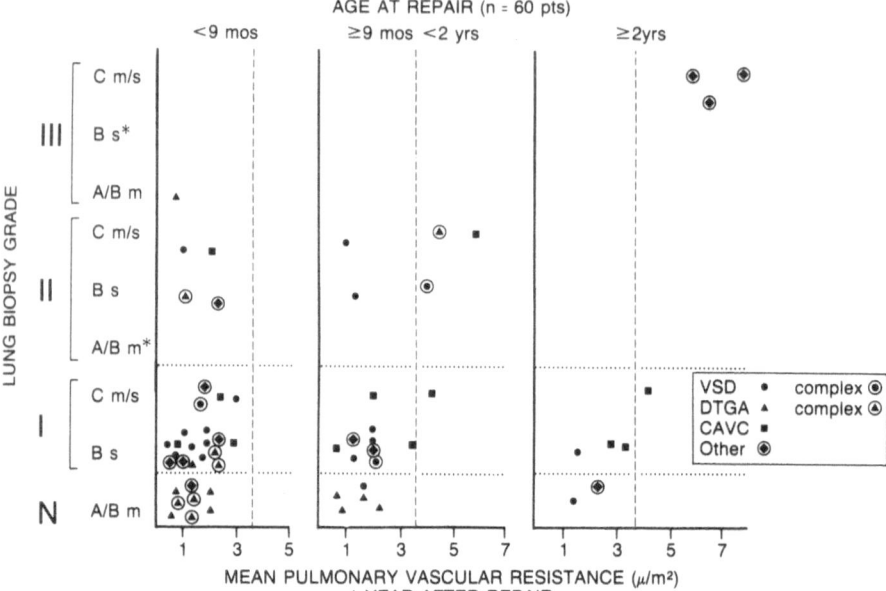

Figure 11. Graph of pulmonary vascular resistance measured one year after corrective surgery in patients with congenital heart defects related to lung biopsy grade. Patients operated upon within the first eight months of life have normal values after surgery regardless of the severity of the lung biopsy grade. (Reproduced with permission (70).)

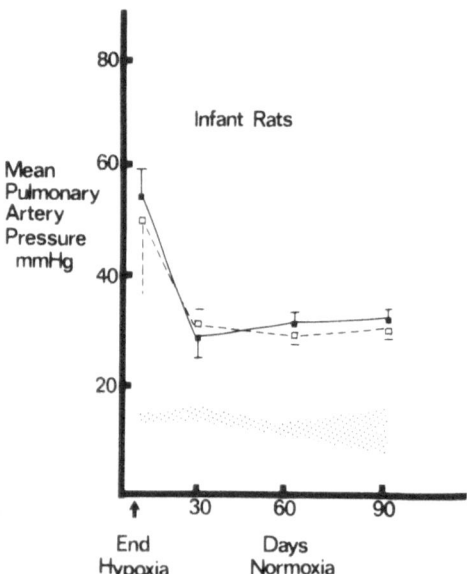

Figure 12A. Graph of mean pulmonary artery pressure values after one month of hypoxia and after 1, 2, and 3 months of recovery in room air in rats exposed from day 8 of life. There is significant residual pulmonary hypertension. Shaded area denotes control range, dotted line = values in female rats; solid line, values in male rats.

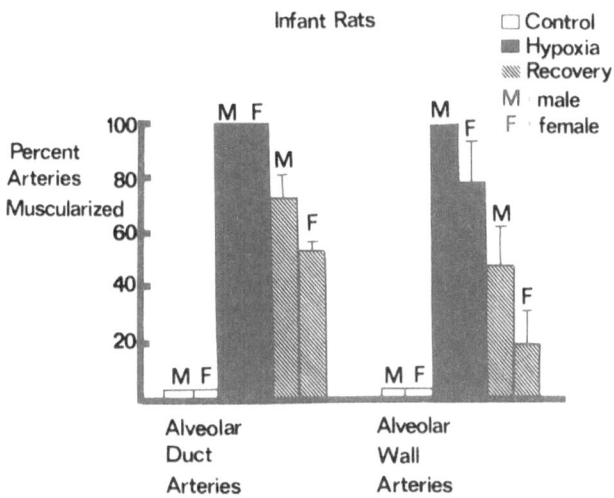

Figure 12B. Graph of alveolar duct and wall arteries abnormally muscularized after one month of hypoxia in the above animals. There is incomplete regression of this structural change in room air.

Chronic hyperoxia (FiO$_2$ 80–100%) results in less of an increase in the muscularity of pulmonary arteries than chronic hypoxia (unpublished observation), but a more striking reduction in arterial concentration (78, 79). Both the degree of regression of hypertrophied smooth muscle and of catch-up growth of arteries depend critically upon the time in development when the stimulus is removed.

THE DEVELOPMENT OF THE MYOCARDIUM

Structural and functional development

In the newborn heart the interventricular septum is first convex to the left, then flat, then, only after a few months, it becomes convex to the right, giving the left ventricle the geometry which favors adaptation to a sudden increase in pressure load (80). Experimental studies show that the myocardium continues to develop structurally for some time after birth (81–83) (Figure 13). Myocardial cells are smaller in the rabbit fetus than in the adult, and within the individual cells there is a higher proportion of noncontractile (mitochondria, etc.) to contractile (myofilaments) mass (81). In newborn compared with adult dogs, myocardial cells are not only smaller but are composed of an assembly of immature and inhomogenous sarcomeres (82, 83). Myocardial cells increase in number only during the first few weeks of life, thereafter they only hypertrophy (84). Jackowski and Kun observed a decrease in polyadenosine diphosphoribosylase activity (85) coincident with this decreased proliferative ability. At this time also Michalak et al.

194

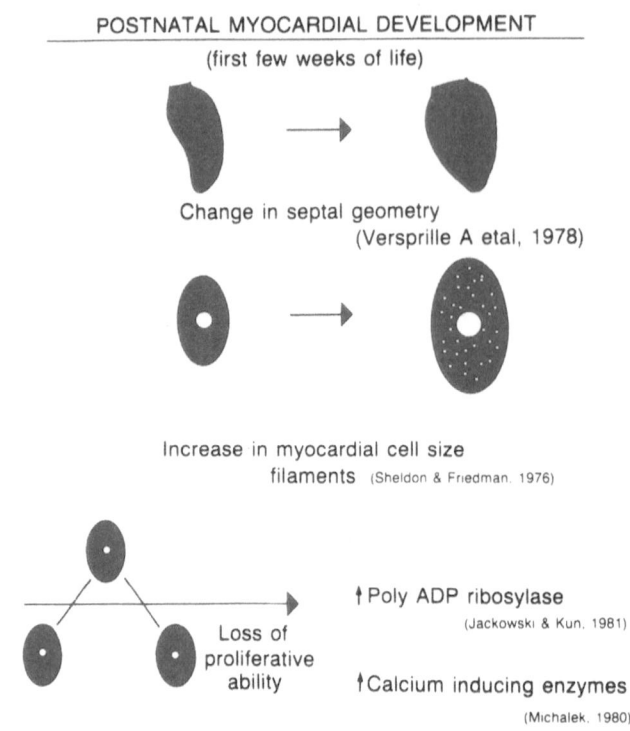

POSTNATAL MYOCARDIAL DEVELOPMENT

(first few weeks of life)

Change in septal geometry
(Versprille A etal, 1978)

Increase in myocardial cell size
filaments (Sheldon & Friedman. 1976)

Loss of
proliferative
ability

↑ Poly ADP ribosylase
(Jackowski & Kun. 1981)

↑ Calcium inducing enzymes
(Michalek. 1980)

Figure 13. Schema depicting changes in myocardial structure shortly after birth.

observed, an induction of the enzymes which govern calcium metabolism (86).

It is logical that the changing structure and biochemistry of the myocardium would be associated with a change in function. Friedman and co-workers observed in lambs, dogs and rabbits that there are differences in the mechanical properties of the myocardium in the fetus, newborn and adult animal (87, 88). The fetus has a stiffer i.e. less compliant ventricle than the adult animal, while the newborn is intermediate. At all muscle lengths along the length tension curve, both active and passive tensions are higher and velocity of shortening less in the fetus and newborn compared with the adult (Figure 14). Thus, while the newborn resting cardiac output per kg body weight is higher than the adult's, the newborn heart is likely functioning at a different point in the Starling curve and this may explain both its inability to handle additional volume loading (89–91), and, in part, its decreased responsivity to inotropic support (92, 93). For example, experimental studies comparing newborn puppies with adult dogs (92) have shown less of an increase in cardiac output in response to isoproterenol, dopamine or dobutamine. Albeit other as yet unexplained factors may also play a role and these include receptor maturation and availability. In addition, neuro-humoral maturation of the heart is important in these responses; from experimental studies in dogs, it appears that the former is not complete at birth but continues

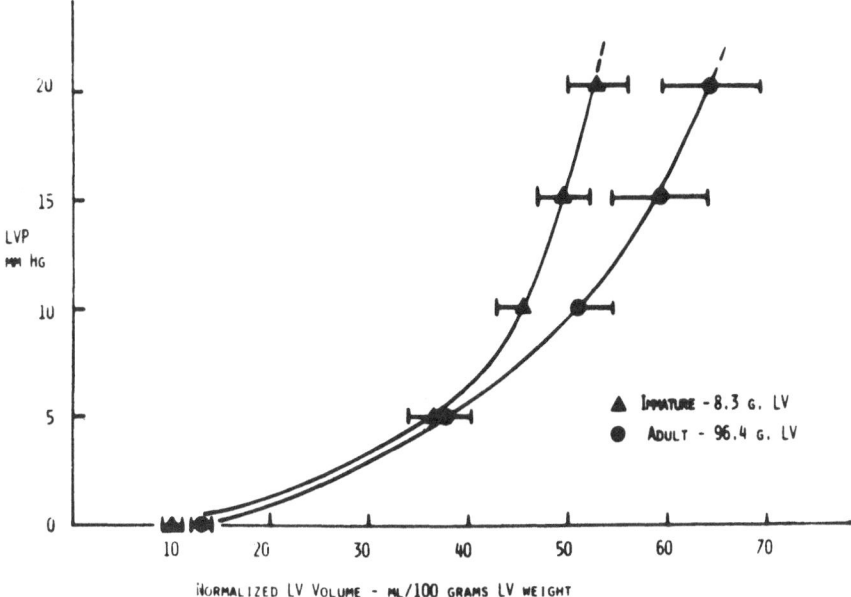

Figure 14. Comparison of pressure volume curves in immature and adult dogs showing the stiffer ventricle in the former. (Reproduced with permission (83).)

to develop thoughout the first six months of life (93). There is histochemical evidence that norepinephrine stores are lower in the fetus than the adult and located mostly in the preterminal nerve trunks rather than in the terminal nerve endings. Also, activity of tyrosine hydroxylase, the norepinephrine-producing enzyme, is less. Thus, the heart demonstrates denervation hypersensitivity to norepinephrine. The parasympathetic system is fully functional in the newborn animal, and gradually becomes the dominant system in the first few months after birth, controlling heart rate and reflex responses to blood pressure.

The functional response of the newborn myocardium to acute stress

'Transient' myocardial ischemia
The newborn ventricle whose structure and geometry does not allow for much compliance would likely respond to an anoxic or metabolic (acidotic, hypoglycemic or hypocalcemic) insult with more severe compromise of ventricular function than the adult ventricle (94). Furthermore, heightened responsivity to circulating catecholamines may result in severe coronary vasoconstriction causing ischemic damage and rarely, tricuspid insufficiency or papillary muscle necrosis and mitral insufficiency. The newborn refractoriness to inotropic support may make this a condition particularly difficult to manage. To further compound

matters, the elevated left atrial pressure resulting from the ventricular dysfunction is a cause of persistent pulmonary hypertension of the newborn, increased right to left shunting and progressive hypoxemia (95).

The structural response of the myocardium to chronic hemodynamic stress

In utero

Chronic hemodynamic stress in utero as a result of left-sided obstruction will, depending upon the level of obstruction, result in either overdevelopment or underdevelopment of the myocardium. For example, the newborn heart which is hypertrophied as a result of critical aortic stenosis, or critical coarctation of the aorta, has a deranged fiber array (96) and an unfavorable myocardial supply–demand ratio (97). The latter may be further compromised by accompanying endocardial fibroelastosis. Patients with mitral stenosis or obstructed total anomalous pulmonary venous drainage have a small left ventricle (98). Both the overdeveloped and underdeveloped ventricle are ill prepared to sustain a compromise in blood supply which may occur during the operative procedure. Delaying surgery, however, will result in further maldevelopment.

Postnatal

Postnatally, the development of intra- or extracardiac left to right shunting in infants with congenital heart defects often adds a volume load to a pressure-overloaded ventricle. The resiliency of either the right or left ventricle will depend to a large extent upon when repair is undertaken (99–102) – the earlier the more likely will there be complete return to normal function and normal response to stress (102).

In infants with cyanotic heart disease high coronary resistance resulting from arterial hypoxemia and hyperviscosity further contributes to the deficit in myocardial oxygenation which results in fibrosis and dysfunction (102).

THE SYSTEMIC VASCULAR BED

Structural development

Experimental studies in dogs and lambs (103–109) have shown that maturation of the sympathetic nervous system and the baroreceptor reflex occurs after birth. Boatman et al. electrically stimulated the hindlimbs of the newborn dog producing a change in vascular resistance dependent upon age; vasodilatation was elicited during the first two weeks of life, vasoconstriction thereafter (103). Further studies demonstrated that peripheral sympathetic fibers develop mostly after birth and reach full maturity at about two months of life (104). This maturational change is associated with a progressive rise in mean systemic blood pressure and with appropriate reflex responses to direct and indirect sympathetic stimulation. In studies by Woods et al. in lambs (105, 196), maturation of neurohumoral control was shown to be responsible for the fall in heart rate from birth, the decrease in resting cardiac output/kg and the rise in systemic arterial pressure (107).

Functional response

In conscious newborn lambs, Manders et al. observed a depressed blood pressure response to vasoconstrictor agents (methexamine, angiotensin II, norepine-phrine) as well as to vasodilator agents (nitroglycerin and isoproterenol) (108, 109) (Figure 15). The decreased response to adrenergic agents may be due to delayed maturation of the sympathetic nervous system. The decreased response to angiotensin II or nitroglycerin may be due to receptor changes as yet un-detected, or the fact that newborn smooth muscle is able to generate less tension than the adult (110). Alternatively, this may represent a dilutional effect, as the blood volume per kg body weight is greater in the newborn than the adult (111).

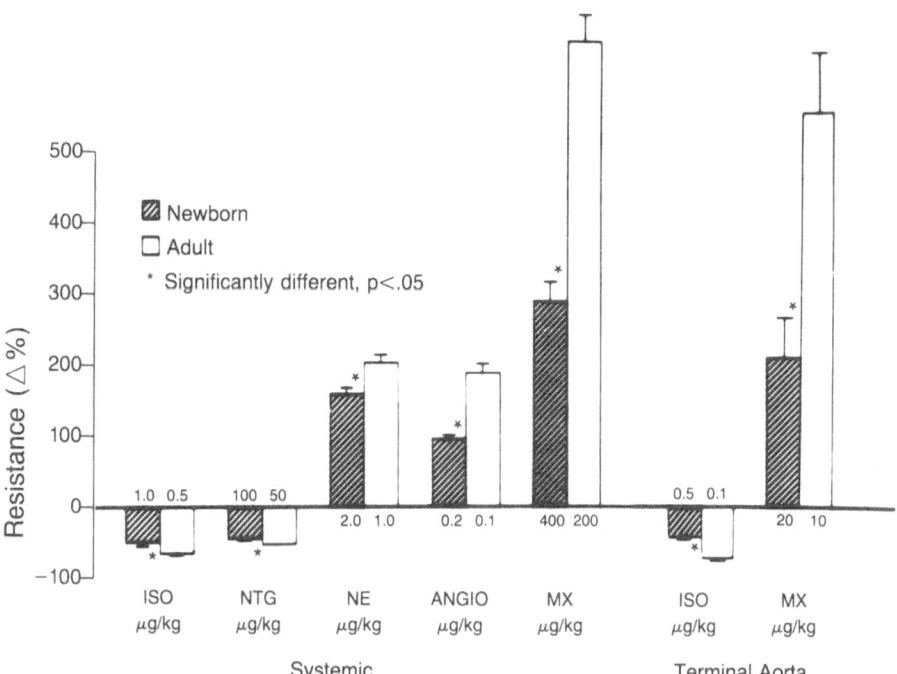

Figure 15. Decreased response to both vasoconstrictor and vasodilator agents in newborn compared to adult lambs. (Reproduced with permission (109).)

198

SUMMARY

It would seem that since maturation of the pulmonary vascular bed, myocardium, and systemic vascular bed is required for an optimum response to stress, the newborn is in a particularly vulnerable position. Current management must therefore aim to alleviate the stress by optimizing myocardial and circulatory support. Finding therapeutic agents which will act optimally within the narrow margins imposed by the newborn circulation should be one goal of current research, hastening structural maturation another, protecting against the malleability of developing structures to chronic hemodynamic stress, a third.

REFERENCES

1. Short DS: The application of arteriography to the pathological study of pulmonary hypertension. In: Adams WR, Veith I (eds), Pulmonary Circulation. Grune and Stratton, New York, pp 233–242, 1959
2. Elliott FM, Reid L: Some new facts about the pulmonary artery and its branching pattern. Clin Radiol 6:196–198, 1965
3. Davies G, Reid L: Growth of the alveoli and pulmonary arteries in childhood. Thorax 25:669–681, 1970
4. Hislop A, Reid L: Pulmonary artery development during childhood: branching pattern and structure. Thorax 28:129–135, 1973
5. Meyrick B, Reid L: Ultrastructural findings in lung material from children with congenital heart defects. Am J Pathol 101:527–537, 1980
6. Rudolph AM, Auld PAM, Golinko RJ, Paul MH: Pulmonary vascular adjustments in the neonatal period. Pediatrics 28:28–34, 1961
7. Haworth SG, Reid L: A morphometric study of regional variation in lung structure in infants with pulmonary hypertension. Br Heart J 40:825–831, 1978
8. Kitiwaga M, Hislop A, Boyden EA, Reid L: Lung hypoplasia in congenital diaphragmatic hernia: a quantitative study of airway, artery and alveolar development. Br J Surg 58:342–346, 1971
9. Hislop A, Reid L: Persistent hypoplasia of the lung following repair of congenital diaphragmatic hernia. Thorax 31:450–455, 1976
10. Bloss RS, Turmen T, Beardmore HE, Aranda JV: Tolazoline therapy for persistent pulmonary hypertension after congenital diaphragmatic hernia repair. J Pediatr 97:984–988, 1980
11. Hardesty RL, Griffith BP, Debski RF, Jeffries MR, Borovetz HS: Extracorporeal membrane oxygenation. Successful treatment of persistent fetal circulation following repair of congenital diaphragmatic hernia. J Thorac Cardiovasc Surg 81:556–563, 1981
12. Hislop A, Hey E, Reid L: The lungs in congenital bilateral renal agenesis and dysplasia. Arch Dis Child 54:32–38, 1979
13. Chamberlain D, Hislop A, Hey E, Reid L: Pulmonary hypoplasia in babies with severe rhesus isoimmunization: a quantitative study. J Pathol 122:43–52, 1977
14. Rendas A, Brown ER, Avery ME, Reid LM: Prematurity, hypoplasia of the pulmonary vascular bed and hypertension: fatal outcome in a ten-month old infant. Am Rev Respir Dis 121:873–880, 1980
15. Goldstein JD, Reid LM: Pulmonary hypoplasia resulting from phrenic nerve agenesis and diaphragmatic amyoplasia. J Pediatr 97:282–287, 1980
16. Riemenschneider TA, Neilson HC, Ruttenberg HD, Jaffe RB: Disturbances of the transitional

circulation: spectrum of pulmonary hypertension and myocardial dysfunction 89:622–625, 1976

17. Lock JE, Fuhrman BP, Epstein ML, Rower RD, Lucas RV: Pulmonary hypertension following neonatal shock. Ped Cardiol 1:109–115, 1979/80

18. Murphy JD, Rabinovitch M, Reid L: Pulmonary vascular pathology in fatal neonatal meconium aspiration. Pediatr Res 15:11–673 (abstract), 1981

19. Rowe RD, Hoffman T: Transient myocardial ischemia of the newborn infant: a form of severe cardiorespiratory distress in fullterm infants. J Pediatr 81:243–250, 1972

20. Peckham GJ, Fox WW: Physiologic factors affecting pulmonary artery pressure in infants with persistent pulmonary hypertension. J Pediatr 93:1005–1010, 1978

21. Lock JE, Olley PM, Coceani F, Swyer PR, Rowe RD: Use of prostacyclin in persistent fetal circulation (letter). Lancet 1:134, 1979

22. Drummond WH, Gregory GA, Heymann MA, Phibbs RA: The independent effects of hyperventilation, tolazoline and dopamine on infants with persistent pulmonary hypertension. J Pediatr 98:603–611, 1981

23. Haworth SG, Reid L: Persistent fetal circulation: newly recognized structural features. J Pediatr 88:614–620, 1976

24. Murphy JD, Rabinovitch M, Goldstein JD, Reid L: The structural basis of persistent pulmonary hypertension of the newborn infant. J Pediatr 98:962–967, 1981

25. McKenzie S, Haworth SG: Occlusion of peripheral pulmonary vascular bed in a baby with idiopathic persistent fetal circulation. Br heart J 46:675–678, 1981

26. Said SI: Metabolic functions of the pulmonary circulation. Circ Res 50:325–333, 1982

27. Ryan VS, Ryan JW: Correlations between the fine structure in the alveolar-capillary unit and its metabolic activities. In: Vane JR, Bankle YS (eds), Metabolic Functions of the Lung, Vol 4: Lenfant C (ed), Lung Biology in Health and Disease. Marcel Dekker, New York, 1977

28. Levin DL, Weinberg AG, Perkin RM: Pulmonary microthrombi syndrome in newborn infants with unresponsive persistent pulmonary hypertension. J Pediatr 102:299–303, 1983

29. Andrew M, Bhogal M, Karpatkin M: Factors XI and XII and prekallikrein in sick and healthy premature infants. New Engl J Med 305:1130–1133, 1981

30. Manchester D, Margolis HS, Sheldon RE: Possible association between maternal indomethacin therapy and primary pulmonary hypertension of the newborn. Am J Obstet Gynecol 126:467–469, 1976

31. Levin DL, Fixler DE, Morriss FC, Tyson J: Morphologic analysis of the pulmonary vascular bed in infants exposed in utero to prostaglandin synthetase inhibitors. J Pediatr 83:964–972, 1978

32. Levin DL, Mills LJ, Weinberg AG: Hemodynamic pulmonary vascular and myocardial abnormalities secondary to pharmacologic constriction of the fetal ductus arteriosus. Circulation 60:360–364, 1979

33. Heymann MA, Rudolph AM: Effects of acetylsalicylic acid on the ductus arteriosus and circulation of fetal lambs in utero. Circ Res 38:418–422, 1976

34. Harker L, Kirkpatrick SE, Friedman WG, Blood CM: Effects of indomethacin on fetal pulmonary circulation. Lab Invest 42:121, 1980

35. Cassin S, Tyler T, Wallis R: The effects of prostaglandin E_1 on fetal pulmonary vascular resistance. Proc Soc Exp Biol Med 148:584–587, 1975

36. Leffler CW, Tyler TL, Cassin S: Response of pulmonary and systemic circulations of perinatal goats to prostaglandin $F_2\alpha$. Can J Physiol Pharmacol 57:167–173, 1979

37. Lock JE, Olley PM, Coceani F, Hamilton F, Doubilet G: Pulmonary and systemic vascular responses to 6-keto PGE_1 in the conscious lamb. Prostaglandins 18:303–309, 1979

38. Cassin S, Todd M, Philips J, Frissinger J, Jordan J, Gibbs C: Effects of prostaglandin D_2 on perinatal circulation. Am J Physiol 240:H755–H760, 1981

39. Starling MB, Neutze J, Elliott RL: Control of elevated pulmonary vascular resistance in neonatal swine with prostacyclin (PGI_2). Prostaglandin Med 3:103–000, 1979

40. Yokochi K, Olley PM, Sideris F, Hamilton F, Huhtanen D, Coceani F: Leukotriene D_4: a potent

vasoconstrictor of the pulmonary and systemic circulations in the newborn lamb. In: Samuelsson B, Paoletti R (eds), Leukotrienes and Other Lipoxygenase Products. Raven Press, New York, pp 211–214, 1982

41. Stenmark KR, James SL, Voelkel NF, Toews WH, Reeves JT, Murphy RC: Leukotriene C_4 and D_4 in neonates with hypoxemia and pulmonary hypertension. New Engl J Med 309–77–80, 1983
42. Lock JE, Hamilton F, Olley PM, Coceani F: The effect of alveolar hypoxia on pulmonary vascular responsiveness in the conscious lamb. Can J Physiol Pharmacol 58:153–159, 1980
43. James LS, Rowe RD: The pattern of response of pulmonary and systemic arterial pressures in newborn and older infants to short periods of hypoxia. J Pediatr 51:5–11, 1957
44. Gilbert RB, Hessler JR, Eitzman DV, Cassin S: Site of pulmonary vascular resistance in fetal goats. J Appl Physiol 32:47–53, 1972
45. Tucker A, McMurtry IF, Reeves JT, Alexander AF, Will DH, Gover RF: Lung vascular smooth muscle as a determinant of pulmonary hypertension at high altitude. Am J Physiol 228:762–767, 1975
46. Cook CD, Drinker PA, Jacobson HN, Levison H, Shang LB: Control of pulmonary blood flow in the foetal and newly born lamb. J Physiol 169:10–29, 1963
47. Rudolph AM, Yuan S: Response of the pulmonary vasculature to hypoxia and H^+ ion concentration changes. J Clin Invest 45:399–411, 1966
48. Cassin S, Dawer GS, Mott JC, Ross BB, Strang LB: The vascular resistance of the foetal and newly ventilated lung of the lamb. J Physiol 171:61–79, 1964
49. Shapiro BJ, Simmons DM, Linde LM: Pulmonary hemodynamics during acute acid–base changes in the intact dog. Am J Physiol 210:1026–1032, 1966
50. Levy AM, Hanson JS, Tabakin BS: Congestive heart failure in the newborn infant in the absence of primary cardiac disease. Am J Cardiol 26:409–415, 1970
51. Fouron JC, Hebert F: The circulatory effects of hematocrit variations in normovolemic newborn lambs. J Pediatr 82:995–1003, 1973
52. Haworth SG, Hislop AA: Adaptation of the pulmonary circulation to extrauterine life in the pig and its relevance to the human infant. Cardiovasc Res 15:108–119, 1981
53. Meyrick B, Reid L: Pulmonary arterial and alveolar development in normal postnatal rat lung. Am Rev Respir Dis 125:468–473, 1982
54. Rendas A, Braithwaite M, Reid L: Growth of the pulmonary circulation in normal pig: structural analysis and aspects of cardiopulmonary function. J Appl Physiol 45:806–817, 1978
55. Meyrick B, Reid L: The effect of chronic hypoxia on pulmonary arteries in young rats. Exp Lung Res 2:257–271, 1981
56. Bland RD, Bressack MA, Haberkern CM, Hansen TN: Lung fluid balance in hypoxic awake newborn lambs and mature sheep. Biol Neonate 38:221–228, 1980
57. Colebatch JHJ, Dawes GS, Goodwin JW: The nervous control of the circulation in the circulation in the fetal and newly expanded lungs of the lamb. J Physiol 178:544–562, 1965
58. Lewis AB, Heymann MA, Rudolph AM: Gestational changes on pulmonary vascular responses in fetal lambs in utero. Circ Res 39:536–541, 1976
59. Silove ED, Gover RF: Effects of alpha adrenergic blockade and tissue catecholamine depletion on pulmonary vascular responses to hypoxia. J Clin Invest 47:274–285, 1968
60. Lock JE, Olley PM, Coceani F: Enhanced beta-adrenergic receptor responsiveness in the hypoxic neonatal pulmonary circulation. Am J Physiol 240:697–703, 1981
61. Newman JH, Souhrada JF, Reeves JT, Arroyave CM, Gover RF: Postnatal changes in response of canine neonatal pulmonary arteries to histamine. Am J Physiol 237:H76–H82, 1979
62. Davidson D, Stalcup SA, Mellins RB: Angiotensin coverting enzyme activity and its modulation by oxygen tension in the guinea pig fetal placental unit. Circ Res 48:286–291, 1981
63. Stalcup SA, Davidson D, Mellins RB: Pulmonary metabolism of vasoactive substances in normal and asphyxiated births. In: Peckham GJ, Heymann MA (eds), Cardiovasular Sequelae of Asphyxia in the Newborn. Report of the Eighty-third Ross Conference on Pediatric Re-

search, Ross Laboratories, Columbus, Ohio, pp 44–51, 1982

64. Rabinovitch M, Grady S, David I, Van Praagh R, Sauer U, Buhlmeyer K, Castaneda AR, Reid L: Compression of intrapulmonary bronchi by abnormally branching pulmonary arteries associated with absent pulmonary valves. Am J Cardiol 50:804–813, 1982

65. Haworth SG, Reid L: Quantitative structural study of pulmonary circulation in the newborn with pulmonary atresia. Thorax 32:129–133, 1977

66. Haworth SG, Reid L: Structural study of the pulmonary circulation in total anomalous pulmonary venous return in early infancy. Br Heart J 39:80–92, 1977

67. Haworth SG, Reid L: Quantitative structural study of pulmonary circulation in the newborn with aortic atresia, stenosis or coarctation. Thorax 32:121–128, 1977

68. Rabinovitch M, Haworth SG, Castaneda AR, Nadas AS, Reid LM: Lung biopsy in congenital heart defects: a morphometric approach to pulmonary vascular disease. Circulation 58:1107–1122, 1978

69. Heath D, Edwards JE: The pathology of hypertensive pulmonary vascular disease. Circulation 18:533–547, 1958

70. Rabinovitch M, Keane JF, Norwood WI, Castaneda AR, Reid L: Vascular structure in lung biopsy tissue correlated with pulmonary hemodynamic findings after repair of congenital heart defects. Circulation 69:655–667, 1984.

71. Jones OOH, Shore DF, Rigby ML, Leijala M, Scallan J, Shinebourne EA, Lincoln JCR: The use of tolazoline hydrochloride as a pulmonary vasodilator in potentially fatal episodes of pulmonary vasoconstriction after cardiac surgery in children. Circulation 64:11–134–139, 1981

72. Addonizio VP Jr, Smith JB, Strauss JF III, Colman RW, Edmunds LM Jr: Thromboxane synthesis and platelet secretion during cardiopulmonary bypass with bubble oxygenator. J Thorac Cardiovasc Surg 79:91–96, 1980

73. Rabinovitch M, Andrew M, Thom H, Williams WG, Trusler GA, Rowe RD, Olley PM, Wilson GJ: Abnormal pulmonary vascular endothelial metabolism of factor VIII in patients with pulmonary hypertension. Circulation 68:111–136 (abstract), 1983

74. Rabinovitch M, Trusler GA, Williams WG, Rowe RD, Olley PM, Cutz E: Pulmonary vascular endothelium and pulmonary hypertension: a correlation of scanning and transmission electron with light microscopy. Circulation 68:111–403 (abstract), 1983

75. Samuelsson B: Leukotrienes and other Lipoxygenase Products. Samuelsson B, Paoletti R (eds). Raven Press, New York, 1982

76. Reid L: Bronchopulmonary dysplasia – pathology. J Pediatr 95:836–841, 1979

77. Rabinovitch M, Gamble WJ, Miettinen OS, Reid L: Age and sex influence on pulmonary hypertension of chronic hypoxia and on recovery. Am J Physiol 240:H62–H72, 1981

78. Frank L, Bucher JR, Roberts RJ: Oxygen toxicity in neonatal and adult animals of various species. J Appl Physiol 45:699–704, 1978

79. Roberts RJ, Weesner KM, Bucher JR: Oxygen-induced alterations in lung vascular development in the newborn rat. Pediatr Res 17:368–375, 1983

80. Versprille A, Jansen JRC, Harinck E, van Nie CF, de Neef: Functional interaction of both ventricles at birth and the changes during the neonatal period in relation to changes of geometry. In: Longo LD, Reneau R (eds), Fetal and Newborn Cardiovascular Physiology. Garland STPM Press, New York, Chapter 16, Vol 1, pp. 399–413, 1978

81. Sheldon CA, Friedman WF, Sybers HD: Scanning electron microscopy of fetal and neonatal lamb cardiac cells. J Mol Cell Cardiol 8:853–862, 1976

82. Urthaler F, Walker AA, Kawamura K, Hefner LL, James TN: Canine atrial and ventricular muscle mechanics studied as a function of age. Circ Res 42:703–713, 1978

83. Spotnitz WD, Spotnitz HM, Truccone NJ, Cottrel TS, Gersony W, Malm JR, Sonnenblick EM: Relation of ultrastructure and function: sarcomere dimensions, pressure–volume curves and geometry of the intact left ventricle of the immature canine heart. Circ Res 44:679–691, 1979

84. Claycomb WC: DNA synthesis and DNA synthesis and DNA enzymes in terminally differen-

tiating cardiac muscle cells. Exp Cell Res 18:111–114, 1979

85. Jackowski G, Kun E: The influence of triiodothyronine on polyadenosine diphosphoribose polymerase and RNA synthesis in cardiocyte nuclei. J Mol Cell Cardiol 14: 65–70, 1982

86. Michalak M, Campbell KP, MacLennan DH: Localization of the high affinity calcium binding protein and an intrinsic glycoprotein in sarcoplasmic reticulum membranes. J Biol Chem 155:1317–1326, 1980

87. Friedman WF, Pool PE, Jacobowitz D, Seagran SC, Braunwald E: Sympathetic innervation of the developing rabbit heart: biochemical and histochemical comparisons of fetal, neonatal and adult myocardium. Circ Res 23:25–32, 1968

88. Friedman WF: The intrinsic physiologic properties of the developing heart. In: Friedman WF, Lesch M, Sonnenblick EH (eds) Neonatal Heart Disease. Grune and Stratton, New York, pp 21–50, 1973

89. Fouron JC, Hebert F: Cardiovascular adaptation of newborn lambs to hypervolemia and polycythemia. Can J Physiol Pharmacol 48:312–320, 1970

90. Klopfenstein HA, Rudolph AM: Postnatal changes in the circulation and responses to volume loading in sheep. Circ Res 42:839–845, 1978

91. Romero TE, Friedman WF: Limited left ventricular response to volume overload in the neonatal period: a comparative study with the adult animal. Pediatr Res 13:910–915, 1979

92. Discoll D, Gillette PD, Fukushige J, Lewis RM, Contant C, Hartley CJ, Entman ML, Schwartz A: Comparison of the cardiovascular action of isoproterenol, dopamine and dolbutamine in the neonatal and mature dog. Pediatr Cardiol 1:307–314, 1980

93. Kralios FA, Millar CR: Functional development of cardiac sympathetic nerves in newborn dogs. Evidence for asymmetrical development. Cardiovasc Res 12:547–554, 1978

94. Rowe RD, Izukawa T, Olley PM, Freedom RF, Swyer PR: Abnormalities of the cardiovascular transition of the newborn: current news on vascular and myocardial responses. In: Goodman MJ (ed), Pediatric Cardiology. Churchill, Livingston, Edinburgh, Chapter 23, pp 236–248, 1981

95. Levin DL, Heymann MA, Ketterman JA, Gregory GA, Phibbs RH, Rudolph AM: Persistent pulmonary hypertension of the newborn infant. J Pediatr 89:626–630, 1976

96. Somerville J, Becu L: Congenital heart disease associated with hypertrophic cardiomyopathy. Johns Hopkins Med J 140:151–162, 1977

97. Hoffman JIE: The myocardial supply–demand ratio. A critical review. Am J Cardiol 58:327–332, 1978

98. Bove KE, Geiser EA, Meyer RA: The left ventricle in anomalous pulmonary venous return. Morphometric analysis in 36 fatal cases in infancy. Arch Pathol 99:522–528, 1975

99. Baylen B, Meyer RA, Korfhagen J, Benzing G, Bubb ME, Kaplan S: Left ventricular performance in the critically ill premature infant with patent ductus arteriosus and pulmonary disease. Circulation 55:182–188, 1977

100. Cordell D, Graham TP Jr, Atwood GF, Boerth RC, Boucek RJ, Bender HW: Left heart volume characteristics following ventricular septal closure in infancy. Circulation 54:417–422, 1976

101. Jamarkani JM, Graham TP Jr, Cavent RVJ: Left ventricular contractile state in children with successfully corrected ventricular sepatal defect. Circulation 46 (Suppl 1):1102–1110, 1972

102. Graham TP Jr, Erath HG Jr, Buckspan GS, Fisher RD: Myocardial anaerobic metabolism during isoprenaline infusion in a cyanotic animal model: possible cause of myocardial dysfunction in cyanotic congenital heart disease. Cardiovasc Res 13:401–406, 1979

103. Boatman DL, Shaffer RA, Dixon RL, Brody MJ: Function of vascular smooth muscle and its sympathetic innervation in the newborn dog. J Clin Invest 44:241–246, 1965

104. Gauthier P, Nadeau P, de Champlain J: The development of sympathetic innervation and the functional state of the cardiovascular system in newborn dogs. Can J Physiol Pharmacol 53:763–776, 1975

105. Woods JR Jr, Dandavino A, Murayama K, Brinkman CR III, Assali NS: Autonomic control of

cardiovascular functions during neonatal development and in adult sheep. Circ Res 40:401–407, 1977

106. Woods JR Jr, Dandavino A, Brinkman CR III, Nuwathid D, Assali NS: Cardiac output changes during neonatal growth. Am J Physiol 234:H520–H524, 1978

107. Magrini F: Hemodynamic determinants of the arterial blood pressure rise during growth in conscious puppies. Cardiovasc Res 12:422–428, 1978

108. Vatner S, Manders WT: Depressed responsiveness of the carotid sinus reflex in conscious newborn animals. Am J Physiol 237:1440–1443, 1979

109. Manders WT, Pagani M, Vatner SF: Depressed responsiveness to vasoconstrictor and dilator agents and baroreflex sensitivity in conscious newborn lambs. Circulation 60:945–955, 1979

110. Pagani M, Mirskey I, Baig H, Manders WT, Kerkhof P, Vatner SF: Effects of age on aortic pressure–diameter and elastic stiffness–stress relations in the unanesthetized sheep. Circ Res 44:420–429, 1979

111. Glantz SA, Kernoff R, Goldman RH: Age related changes in ouabain pharmacology. Ouabain exhibits a different volume distribution in adult and young dogs. Circ Res 39:407–414, 1976

INDEX